Medical Handbook

Medical Handbook

A Consumer Guide for Navigating the Medical System

Gregory G. Billy, M.D.

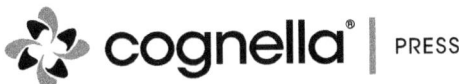

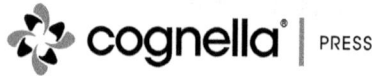

www.cognella.com   800-200-3908

Contents

PREFACE   vii

INTRODUCTION: HOW DID WE GET HERE:
THE HISTORY OF MEDICINE   ix

1.   MEDICAL EDUCATION AND TRAINING   1

2.   MEDICAL AND SURGICAL SPECIALTIES   11

3.   INPATIENT VERSUS OUTPATIENT MEDICINE   23

4.   SELECTING AND NAVIGATING PHYSICIANS'
     OFFICES   31

5.   TESTING AND DIAGNOSES   41

6.   GUIDE TO PRESCRIPTIONS   53

7.   NUTRITION AND HEALTH   65

8.   EXERCISE AND RELATED TOPICS   77

9.   MENTAL HEALTH AND RELATED THERAPIES   85

10. MARIJUANA   97

11. SEXUAL HEALTH   107

12. INSURANCE   121

13. THE INTERNET AND THE WORLD OF MEDICINE   131

14. LONG-TERM CARE AND END-OF-LIFE ISSUES   145

Preface

This book is written for the purpose of educating and enlightening the consumer, aspiring physician, or allied health professional on a number of important topics in medicine. I have practiced as a physician for the past 20-plus years and during my many thousand interactions with patients it is apparent that most patients are not knowledgeable in regards to the healthcare continuum, medical and insurance systems. Patients *do* want to learn but may not know where to turn to for good medical information.

With a goal of educating consumers to medical information, I have taught HPA 057 course at Pennsylvania State University since 2014, educating more than two thousand students in regards to health choices, insurance, and the world of medicine. Student feedback from the course has been overwhelmingly positive and inspiring. I have focused on efforts to bring this information to the general public.

This book is written to serve as such a resource. I hope that you will find this book easy to read and concise but comprehensive in its coverage. The focus on each chapter is to provide the consumer with a basic overview of the topic, explain how it can directly affect you, and provide additional reliable resources for further study.

In medicine, physicians like to provide other physicians with "clinical pearls." These pearls are bits of important information that have been discovered, learned, and utilized with good results. The end of each chapter will list clinical "pearl" information to further expand and highlight points of the chapter, with the expectation that it may enhance your health in a positive way.

—Gregory G. Billy, MD

Introduction

How Did We Get Here: The History of Medicine

We are blessed to live in the United States and tend to take a lot of our fortune for granted. This includes the state of medicine and our medical care. There are likely choices to make between competing medical centers, insurance carriers, and well-trained physicians. In addition, most medical facilities are a few minutes away and easily accessible, but this was not always the case. Just over two hundred years ago there were only two hospitals in the United States. Yes, you read that correctly, two. The first hospital was in Philadelphia, founded in 1755, followed by New York Hospital in 1771.

By 1873 the United States had about 180 hospitals. Even though the number of hospitals increased during those one hundred years, the care at hospitals cannot compare to today's standards. Early hospitals were not organized and had little to offer in terms of specialty care. Most hospitals only had operating rooms for surgery. Unfortunately, physicians and medical caregivers at that time also had little to no understanding of infection, and diseases would spread quickly among patients. Hospitals were sadly breeding grounds for sickness and death. Mortality rates in the early hospitals approached 90%. Additionally, physicians were neither affiliated with nor an integral part of hospitals, as they are today. Physicians would administer their care at the home of the patient during house calls. Technology (stethoscope) at that time was very limited and could fit into the doctor's bag.

A significant factor that advanced health care was a growing understanding of infection. In the late 19th century, Joseph Lister noted that nearly 50% of amputation patients died from sepsis. A few years later he learned of Louis Pasteur's theory of infections caused by microorganisms. Lister began using carbolic acid as an antiseptic to reduce bacterial contamination and was able to reduce the mortality rate in his surgical unit to 15%. This significantly improved the care that was being provided at hospitals. Another factor that helped bring significant improvements in the American hospital system was the Civil War. The war was costly to our country in both injuries and casualties. Given the significant number of injuries and the desire to get the injured soldiers back to the fronts, hospitals needed to improve both their care and organization.

Hospitals continued to improve, and the relationship with physicians also changed. By the late 1800s, hospitals became essential to the practice of medicine and physicians. Technologies and outcomes improved significantly, and physicians began associating with hospitals. They began to admit their patients to hospitals for care. Physicians would follow the patients in the hospital for better outcomes, rather than solely providing home visits. Paramount to receiving better care in the hospital was the care provided by the nurses during a patient's stay. Nursing was unspecialized in the mid-1800s. There were no standards for education or certification. Hospitals may have been staffed by caring individuals, but the modern-day standards of nursing did not exist. Florence Nightingale founded the first nursing school at St. Thomas' Hospital in London. The nursing school would address educational and professional standards that are in place today.

Technology has continued to improve our ability to both provide and administer care. Advancements in medications, diagnostic equipment, and surgical techniques have enabled us to provide the care today that most Americans take for granted.

Chapter 1

Medical Education and Training

A sk the average person how many years of education and training it takes to become a physician and most will answer "a lot." When provided with the correct answer, some will be surprised at the total number of years of training. This chapter will briefly discuss how medical education was shaped in the United States as well as answer how many years it takes to become a doctor. In addition, the content will help the consumer become more familiar with what the medical training entails as well as explain the terms intern, resident, and fellow.

Early Medical Education

During the 1600s and 1700s, most colonial Americans intending to practice medicine would serve as an apprentice for an already established physician. In Europe, small groups of physicians would create proprietary medical schools.[1] The wealthy would travel to Europe, typically Great Britain, to receive training either at a proprietary school or hospital. The larger cities, London, Edinburgh, and Paris, offered medical schools with the advantage of learning at these larger hospitals. Others entered the medical profession more directly by establishing a reputation as a healer or by selling curatives.

During the mid- to late 1700s, medical schools were established in the United States. By 1820 there were 13 medical schools in the United States.[2] The first medical school in the country was the University of Pennsylvania. Once schools were established, they began to develop a curriculum; early training consisted of eight to ten months of class lectures followed by a period of serving as an apprentice, which is similar to the modern-day education of physicians. Toward the late 1800s medical schools developed a curriculum that was more rigorous, as medical knowledge expanded and became more grounded in science.[3] However, there was significant variation between the education and training provided at the various schools.

Flexner Report

Due to this variation medical school education was extensively evaluated in 1910 by Abraham Flexner. He was an educator and member of the research staff of the Carnegie Foundation. He surveyed all 155 medical and osteopathic educational institutions in the United States and Canada and published a comprehensive report of the state of medical education.

Flexner concluded that the education offered by medical institutions was substandard, that there were too many institutions, and that freestanding educational institutions were unable to provide a quality level of education. His report further recommended that medical schools have minimum admission standards to include a high school education and at least two years of studies at the college level. Additionally, the report recommended that medical schools should be four years in duration: two years of basic sciences and two years of clinical education. As a result of the report's recommendations, between 1910 and 1935 more than half of all American medical schools merged or closed. The majority of the affected schools were osteopathic schools.

Of the 66 surviving medical schools in 1935, 57 were part of a university. It is somewhat remarkable that more than one hundred years later the *Flexner Report* still serves as the basis for medical education in the United States today.

Medical School

Today there are 171 medical schools in the United States. The majority of which (84 percent) are found in the Eastern and Central time zones. Acceptance into medical school is extremely competitive and once accepted it is very expensive. According to the Association of American Medical Colleges the average cost of a public medical school is $35,704 per year and $57,194 per year at a private medical school. There are two subtypes of medical schools: allopathic and osteopathic. Osteopathic medical schools originated in and are unique to the United States. Allopathic schools will confer the doctor of medicine (MD) degree and the osteopathic schools the doctor of osteopathy (DO) degree.

Allopathic schools have a more competitive admissions process than osteopathic schools. Graduates of either school are doctors after completing a four-year medical education program and licensure. Allopathic graduates will be licensed after successfully passing the three-step United States Medical Licensure Examination (USMLE). The National Board of Osteopathic Medical Examiners administers a three-step examination COMLEX-USA to osteopathic graduates for licensure. The allopathic approach focuses on diagnosis and treatment based on a patient's symptoms. The osteopathic approach is a holistic integrative approach treating the patient as a whole person. Osteopaths also train in osteopathic manipulative treatment (OMT), a hands-on approach to treatment. Osteopathic schools produce around 20 percent and allopathic schools about 80 percent of graduating physicians each year.

Medical schools consist of a four-year program. Traditionally, the first two years are spent in labs and classrooms and the last two years in hospitals and clinics. There has been a recent emphasis to increase the medical students' clinical exposure during the first two years of school. During the first year of school the classes include anatomy, physiology, histology, and biochemistry. The second year emphasizes clinical sciences focusing on pathology, microbiology, and pharmacology. In the third year students will begin clinical rotations, spending time on the floors and assisting the medical team in evaluating patients and learning treatment approaches. Most clinical rotations will last between four and eight weeks, giving students a broad exposure to the various disciplines of medicine. During the fourth and final year of medical school, students continue clinical rotations and have opportunities to do elective clinical rotations. The elective rotations are usually in areas that students would like to pursue in a postgraduate program or residency upon graduation from medical school. The entire four-year experience is at times both physically and emotionally challenging and is outlined in table 1.1.

TABLE 1.1   MEDICAL SCHOOL EDUCATION

Year 1, basic sciences: Anatomy, physiology, histology, biochemistry

Year 2, clinical sciences: Pathology, microbiology, pharmacology

Year 3, clinical rotations: Medicine, pediatrics, surgery, ob-gyn

Year 4, clinical rotations: Neurology, emergency medicine, and clinical electives

Postgraduate Education

During their fourth and final year of medical school, prospective doctors will begin applying for postgraduate training positions. These positions are known as internships and residencies. All medical students receive very similar training in medical school. Internships and residencies are the time when physicians gravitate toward a particular medical specialty. What influences which specialty a physician will further train in? Sometimes it is a unique medical student-patient experience that influences which specialty one will chose. Often it may be influenced by a particular instructor-attending physician or senior resident who may influence the choice of specialty. Other times the specialty may be influenced by a family member who is a physician. Certain specialties are better suited to a certain personality type. It is during residency training that different postgraduate skills will emerge and physicians will specialize into various fields.

The Match

Fourth-year medical students will apply to different residency programs, similar to the process of applying to medical schools. The residency program may grant them an interview based on their medical school transcripts, national board scores (USMLE or COMLEX-USA), and letters of recommendation from current medical school professors. The interviews will be scheduled between the medical students and the prospective residency program. The interviews are similar to the medical school interview. The different training programs will provide prospective residents with a tour of the facility, highlighting the positive and unique aspects of their training program. Larger academic and teaching hospitals will have more slots for residents as well as a greater variety of programs. The programs may also be staffed by leading physicians in their particular field. Smaller hospitals with fewer total positions may offer a better opportunity for more hands-on training opportunities. For example, neurologic problems in a larger training program will be seen by a neurology resident or service, while at a smaller hospital these patients would be cared for by the internal medicine resident. Medical students will need to determine which program is best for them based on reputation, training, and location.

After interviewing at a number of residency training programs at their own expense, medical students will then make a list of these programs and rank them in order of preference, based on their desire to train at each particular program. For a nominal fee, students will submit their rank list to the National Resident Matching Program (the Match). The residency programs will also rank medical students based on their preferences and provide their rank lists to the Match.

Match Day

The rank lists are submitted by both medical students and residency programs in January and February, and the results are revealed during match day. Typically in mid-March, medical students will be able to check the status of their match and find out if they matched a program they had ranked. If they did not match, they will be able to get a list of programs that did not fill their internship/residency slots and work on contacting those programs for a residency position. This process is known as the "scramble."

The medical schools will likely have a match day celebration, and all fourth-year medical students will be together. The students will open their appointment letter at the same time to learn of their future destinations. This is another milestone in the education of a physician. It is a unique event, since the soon-to-be physicians will then know the direction for their life for the next three to seven years. The match results often contain surprises that can be both positive and negative. Students may match into a program that they did not think they could get into or into one they wish they had not gotten in to.

Internship

Following medical school, newly graduated physicians will enter a postgraduate training program. Certain residencies that are specialized will have physicians do a year of internship training. Other training programs will not have the physician do an internship, also known as postgraduate year 1 (PGY-1). The *internship* is also known as a transitional or preliminary year. Internships offer a broad exposure to the different aspects of internal medicine or to the different aspects of surgery and are one year in length. Physicians in training are paid during their internship. This also marks the first time that new doctors are responsible for patient care. However, all care is done within a team structure, with interns reporting to higher-trained residents and attending physicians.

Residency

Training programs to provide physicians with more specialized training in certain subspecialties are known as *residencies*. They can vary in length and are listed in table 1.2. Residency programs are accredited by the Accreditation Council for Graduate Medical Education (ACGME), a private organization that sets the standards for graduate medical programs in the United States. The ACGME ensures the programs meet the quality standards of the specialty. Residency training is intense and the hours can be incredibly long. Since 2003 there have been restrictions limiting the number of work hours per week and per shift. Currently, the workweek is capped at eighty hours. First-year residents are not permitted to work more than a 16-hour shift, but this will likely be increased to a 24-hour shift, similar to the limits for other residents. The limits are in place for both patient and resident safety.

During residency training the resident physician will work in a team structure. The team will likely include an intern, junior resident, senior resident, and an attending physician. The responsibilities of residents will increase with their years of training or training level. According to the American Association of Medical Colleges, the starting median salary of a first-year resident or intern is about $53,500. The salaries will typically increase by about $2,000 for each additional year of residency training.

TABLE 1.2 LENGTH OF RESIDENCY TRAINING

Years	Program
3	Family medicine, internal medicine, pediatrics, and emergency medicine
4	Obstetrics and gynecology, pathology, and psychiatry
3, plus PGY-1	Anesthesiology, dermatology, neurology, ophthalmology, and physical medicine and rehabilitation
4, plus PGY-1	Radiology and radiation oncology
5	General surgery, orthopedic surgery, otolaryngology, and plastic surgery
6	Neurological surgery

Following residency, physicians will typically choose either to enter practice or subspecialize further by completing a fellowship.

Fellowship

Following residency, physicians may choose to subspecialize in their field by completing a *fellowship*. Fellowships are typically an additional one to two years of training. Examples include an interventional fellowship in cardiology to get additional training and experience with cardiac catheterizations, a sports medicine fellowship for family practice residents who want to tailor their future practice toward athletic medicine, or a micrographic surgery and dermatologic oncology fellowship in dermatology to gain additional experience in melanoma removal. Not all physicians will choose to do fellowships, as this will add another one to two years to their total years of training.

The answer to the question of how many years of schooling and training it takes to become a physician can vary according to the specialty of the physician and is outlined in table 1.3.

TABLE 1.3   PHYSICIAN EDUCATIONAL TIMELINE

College	Medical School	Internship (if not included in residency)	Residency	Fellowship	Total Years
4	4	(1)	3–6	1–2	11–16

CLINICAL PEARL

Getting accepted into medical school is quite competitive, and the number of applicants for a select number of slots is significant. At first glance the statistics can seem incredibly daunting. For example, the Pennsylvania State University College of Medicine recently received 9,449 applications for only 149 slots. This, mathematically, is a 1.57 percent matriculation rate.

However, keep in mind that the average number of schools that an applicant applies to is 14. So that means if one is accepted, the applicant can only attend 1/14, which equates to 7 percent. According to the most recent AAMC data, the overall acceptance rate is 32 percent. If it is your dream to be a physician, do not let the statistics overwhelm you.

Resources

Accreditation Council for Graduate Medical Education: This website is the home site for ACGME; they accredit residency and fellowship programs to ensure academic standards: http://www.acgme.org

American Association of Colleges of Osteopathic Medicine: Website for osteopathic (DO) physicians. This site serves as a central site for application to osteopathic medical schools, for education for the public, and for a resource for osteopathic physicians: http://www.aacom.org/

Association of American Medical Colleges: Website for allopathic (MD) physicians. This site serves as a central site for application to allopathic medical schools, its members are 151 accredited U.S. and 17 accredited Canadian medical schools, nearly all major teaching hospitals and health systems. It serves as a resource for those considering applying to medical school: http://www.aamc.org/

Association of American Medical Colleges: Home of the academic oversight of medical schools and major teaching hospitals, with a link to specific resident physician salaries: https://www.aamc.org/data/stipend/

National Board of Osteopathic Medical Examiners: Website of the national credentialing examination of osteopathic physicians. This site contains information of the testing and administration of the COMLEX-USA certification examination: http://www.nbome.org

National Resident Matching Program: Home of the residency match program; when and where to apply and details of the match process are answered at this site: http://www.nrmp.org

United States Medical Licensure Examination: Website of the national credentialing examination of allopathic physicians. This site contains information of the testing and administration of the USMLE, the test for medical licensure in the United States: http://www.usmle.org/

Endnotes

1. Elizabeth Fee, "The First American Medical School: The formative years." *The Lancet* 385, no. 9981 (2015): 1940-1.
2. William G., Rothstein, *American Medical Schools and the Practice of Medicine: A History* (New York: Oxford University Press, 1987).
3. Kenneth Ludmerer, *Time to Heal: American Medical Education from the Turn of the Century to the Era of Managed Care* (New York: Oxford University Press, 1999).

Chapter 2

Medical and Surgical Specialties

Today medicine is very specialized and very different than when your grandparents went to one doctor for most "if not all" of their medical needs. About half of all physicians specialize in a specific type of medicine. This changed due to advances in technology as well as our increase in understanding of science, the human body, and disease. Less than 100 years ago all that we knew about medicine was summarized in a three hundred-page book that was filled with more anecdotal tales than science. Today, internal medicine textbooks fill two 1,200-page volumes with information. As a result, medicine has relied more on specialists to provide medical care. This chapter serves as a who's who in medicine guide to educate the consumer on the various medical and surgical specialties.

Generalist is the term to describe a physician who is broadly trained in primary care services and may include family physicians, internists, or pediatricians. The term *specialist* describes a physician who specializes during his or her residency training or further subspecializes by doing an additional fellowship. Choosing to be a generalist or a specialist is typically done in the third year of medical school, when the student will decide on a residency training program following medical school. The main decision point involves deciding to perform or not to perform surgeries. Typically, surgeries are only performed by physicians trained in surgical-related residency programs.

Generalist

A family physician is a generalist who completes a residency training program of three years. The family physician is trained to take care of the entire family, children and adults. Training can also involve gynecology and obstetrics. Depending on geographic location, the family physician may care for pregnant patients and deliver babies (usually in the Western United States). The family physician may also be known as the primary care physician (PCP) or the gate keeper. This term refers to their role with certain insurance programs to provide necessary referrals for their patients to various specialties. They are typically involved with the initial work-up of the patient. This initial work-up may involve ordering various diagnostic tests and referrals to specialists if treatments are beyond their scope of practice. Recently, the position of the PCP is moving toward an outpatient practice with less inpatient coverage of admitted patients.

An internist is another example of a generalist. Internists complete a three-year residency program. Their training will focus on the care of an adult. They can also serve as one's PCP and will begin the initial work-up of a patient. They refer less to a specialist and initiate the treatment for common diseases and problems. Historically, internists have admitted their patients to hospitals for necessary care. There has been a shift more toward an exclusive outpatient practice. Their patients are still admitted to a hospital but may be followed by a *hospitalist*. They are physicians who are trained in taking care of hospitalized patients during their stay in a hospital. The hospitalist may cover the patient in the intensive care unit, telemetry unit, or regular medical floor. They work 12-hour shifts caring for their patients and are employed by the hospital.

A pediatrician is a generalist who is trained in the medical care of children. Pediatricians classically care for patients under the age of 18. The care of a child is distinctly different than caring for an adult. Children have different medical issues and concerns than adults; their treatments also differ in both approach and dosing of medications. Additionally, caring for sick children can be an emotionally trying experience. Seeing a sick or ill child can be quite sobering and it requires the physician to have a certain personality type. Further complicating their care may be the child's inability to speak or to adequately communicate their symptoms. Difficult parents can further present additional challenges. The length of training is three years and various fellowships are available to further subspecialize in the care of children.

General Surgery

In medical school physicians in training will decide to follow a path of medicine or a surgical path following graduation from medical school. Similar to generalists and specialists in medicine, there are generalists and specialists in surgery. General surgery is a five-year residency that is completed following medical school. General surgeons are trained to cover a broad area of diseases in most areas of the body that require surgery. They are also trained in the diagnosis and treatment of patients before, during, and after their surgeries. General surgeons will be trained in surgery involving the abdomen, breasts, and skin. Surgeries involving the brain, spine, thoracic region, and bones will typically be performed by specialists in their fields.

General surgeons will commonly remove infected appendixes and gall bladders. The removal of a gall bladder is known as a cholecystectomy. The gall bladder is removed secondary to infection or accumulation of stones in its wall or duct. The procedure to remove a gall bladder can be done either via an open approach or a laparoscopic one. The open approach is the traditional method; it involves making a 3–5-inch incision in the abdomen to gain access to the organ. The recovery is typically longer, but the complication rate is lower than the laparoscopic approach. The laparoscopic approach uses a laparoscope. This is a device for visualization of the abdominal cavity. Three small 1-inch or smaller incisions are used to permit the scopes to enter the abdominal cavity. Light, devices for visualization, and tools are used to remove the organ. The use of scopes to perform surgeries has become the standard of care for the majority of operations and procedures.

Specialists

Specialists are typically named according the field of study; *ologist* is a suffix that typically denotes a particular field of science or an expert. The field of study is the prefix, and there are typically both medical and surgical specialists for the specific organ systems of the body. Examples are listed in table 2.1.

TABLE 2.1 COMMON SPECIALTIES

Cardio: Heart	Neuro: Brain and nerves
Derm: Skin	Opthalmo: Eyes
Endo: Glands	Pulmo: Lungs
Gastro: Stomach/digestive tract	Path: Disease

Heart
Cardiologist

A cardiologist is a specialist who treats the heart and heart-related problems. Cardiologists first complete a three-year internal medicine residency and then a three-year cardiology fellowship. During the fellowship training they learn to manage various heart-related issues including coronary artery disease, heart failure, or irregular heart rates known as arrhythmias. Some may choose to get additional training and subspecialize by doing a second subspecialty fellowship for an additional two years. The subspecialty training is offered in cardiac catherizations, heart failure, and heart arrhythmias. Cardiologist, based on their training, can treat patients either noninvasively or invasively.

Noninvasive cardiologists will focus on the medical management of disease. Prescribing medications can help reduce heart-related problems. The invasive cardiologist will be proficient in procedures to treat heart disease. These procedures include cardiac catherizations and pacemaker implantation.

Cardiothoracic Surgeon

Cardiothoracic surgeons are surgical specialists who perform surgery on the heart and repair adjacent vessels of the heart. Cardiothoracic surgeons will complete a five-year general surgery residency and an additional three-year residency in cardiothoracic surgery. During their specialty training they may focus on valve replacements, ventricular assist devices, and endoscopic techniques.

Lungs

Pulmonologist

A pulmonologist is a specialist who treats lung and breathing-related issues. Pulmonologists will complete a three-year internal medicine residency and then complete a two-year pulmonary fellowship. It is during the fellowship years they learn to manage respiratory-related conditions. Common lung conditions include asthma, chronic obstructive pulmonary disease (COPD), and infections of the lungs. Pulmonologists will also perform and interpret pulmonary function tests to better understand the capacity and function of the lungs as well as prescribe medications and inhalers to improve breathing.

Pulmonologists will also perform bronchoscopies. A bronchoscopy involves inserting a flexible tube and camera into the trachea (wind pipe) and visualizing the bronchus and proximal lung tissues. During this procedure a tissue sample or biopsy may be taken to investigate a mass in this area.

Thoracic Surgeon

Thoracic surgeons are surgical specialists who perform surgery on the organs of the chest. Thoracic surgeons will complete a five-year general surgery residency and an additional three-year residency in thoracic surgery, which may include cardiothoracic procedures. The thoracic surgeon will focus on diseases of the chest including surgical treatment of lung diseases, tumors of the lung and chest wall, and chest reconstruction following trauma. They are skilled in both open and endoscopic techniques.

Kidneys

Nephrologist

A nephrologist is a specialist who treats diseases related to the kidneys. Nephrologists complete a three-year internal medicine residency and then complete a two- to three-year nephrology fellowship. Disease of the kidney and kidney failure are the main focus of a nephrologist. They will also manage dialysis treatments for patients in renal or kidney failure.

Urologist

A urologist is a surgical specialist who completes a one-year residency in general surgery and then a four-year training program in urology. Urologists are surgeons who treat both males and females for problems of the urinary tract including the kidneys, bladder, and urinary tract infections. In addition, they also treat concerns related to the male reproductive organs, more specifically cancers of the prostate or testicles.

Stomach

Gastroenterologist

A gastroenterologist is a specialist who treats diseases related to the digestive system (from the mouth to the rectum). Gastroenterologists will complete a three-year internal medicine residency and then a three-year fellowship. The fellowship will emphasize subspecialty training of diseases of the gastrointestinal (GI) tract. During this time, the gastroenterologist will become proficient in performing invasive procedures to directly visualize the lining of the GI tract. One procedure is the endoscopy, which is an invasive procedure to visualize the esophagus and stomach. The other is a colonoscopy, which is an invasive procedure to visualize the rectum and large intestine. The procedures are done to evaluate the presence of masses or tumors as well as areas of bleeding. Gastroenterologists will also medically treat inflammatory issues of the bowels and heartburn or reflux issues. Cancers of the gastrointestinal tract are addressed by the general surgeon.

Brain and Nerves

Neurologist

Neurologists are physicians who specialize in the treatment of diseases related to the nervous system. A neurologist will complete a four-year residency. The training will focus of diagnosing and treating diseases of the central nervous system (brain and spinal cord) and the peripheral nervous system (nerves of the body). Neurologists will perform procedures including electrodiagnostic studies (nerve and muscle tests), EEG studies, and sleep studies. In addition, they will also medically manage diseases of the central nervous system, Parkinson's disease, seizures, and multiple sclerosis (MS).

Neurosurgeon

Neurosurgeons are surgeons who specialize in the treatment of the nervous system. Neurosurgeons will complete a seven-year residency. They specialize in the treatment and removal of brain/spinal tumors, treating hydrocephalus (swelling of the ventricles of the brain), and removing brain hemorrhages (bleeds). They may place a shunt in the brain to remove the increased fluid seen with hydrocephalus. They may also need to perform a craniotomy or drill holes in the skull to relieve pressure of the brain following a bleed or hemorrhage. They are typically held in high esteem among medical professionals given their extensive training, level of patient commitment, and on-call requirements.

Diabetes

Endocrinologist

Endocrinologists are specialists who treat diseases related to the glands of the body. They will complete a three-year internal medicine residency and then complete a two- to three-year endocrinology fellowship. The fellowship will focus on the diagnosis and treatment of hormone disorders/imbalances caused by the endocrine glands. The most commonly treated condition is the control of elevated blood glucoses (sugars), known as diabetes mellitus. The development of Type 2 diabetes is closely related to obesity and unfortunately has been on the rise in the United States over the past two decades.

Ears, Nose, and Throat

Otolaryngologist

Otolaryngologists are surgeons who specialize in the treatments of the ears, nose, neck, and throat. Otolaryngologists complete a five-year residency in otolaryngology. These surgeons are commonly referred to as ENTs (ear, nose, and throat). Otolaryngology specialists are trained in procedures related to the ear, nose, sinuses, larynx, head, and neck. They commonly perform tonsillectomies, sinus surgeries, and nasal septum surgeries including septoplasties and cancers resections involving the head and neck. They commonly also perform myringotomies, a procedure to install tubes in one's ear drums to allow drainage of recurrent ear infections.

Mental Health

Psychiatrist

Psychiatrists are physicians who specialize in the diagnosis and treatment of mental disorders. A psychiatrist will complete a four-year residency. The focus on their training is to evaluate patients to determine whether their symptoms are the result of a physical illness, a combination of physical and mental, or a strictly psychiatric illness. Psychiatrists can easily subspecialize in various areas including addiction disorders, child and adolescent psychiatry, geriatric psychiatry, and forensic psychiatry. Psychiatrists may work closely with counselors and psychologists to help treat patients. The main difference between a psychiatrist and a psychologist is the former is a medical doctor who can prescribe medications while the latter is unable to prescribe medications.

Skin

Dermatologist

Dermatologists are physicians who specialize in the treatment of disorders of the skin. Dermatologists will complete a four-year residency. They become proficient in the identification and treatment of skin disorders, growths, and cancers. Dermatologists will perform procedures to remove skin lesions, typically removing them via cutting or freezing.

Plastic and Reconstructive Surgeon

Plastic and reconstructive surgeons specialize in microsurgeries and reconstruction. They spend six years in a residency specializing in these skills. They are exposed to complex reconstruction surgeries involving the breast, head, neck, abdominal wall, and peripheral nerve procedures during their training. The plastics aspect of their field typically involves procedures done for cosmetic purposes including breast augmentation and facial surgeries. The elective procedures are rarely covered by insurance and patients will need to pay for these procedures from their own private funds. The reconstructive aspect of their field will involve scar revision, cleft lip/palate repair, burn skin repair/revision, and reconstruction of the breasts following their removal for a cancer (mastectomy). Additional skills of a plastic surgeon may involve reconstruction of injured nerves.

Musculoskeletal System

Physiatrist

Physiatrists are physicians who specialize in the treatment of musculoskeletal diseases and disorders that lead to a change or decline in function that may benefit from treatments directed at rehabilitation. Physiatrists will complete a four-year residency, commonly known as physical medicine and rehabilitation (PM&R). The physical medicine portion can be thought of as nonoperative orthopedics addressing pain and problems related to the musculoskeletal system. The rehabilitation aspect focuses on directing a team of therapists working to have a patient recover from a disorder causing a significant change in function. Stroke, spinal cord injuries, traumatic brain injuries, and amputations are examples of such disorders. Additionally, physiatrists also perform electrodiagnostic studies or may perform spinal injections. Injections may address pain and decreased function secondary to disc herniations and spinal arthritis.

Orthopedic Surgeon

Orthopedic surgeons specialize in the treatment of bone and musculoskeletal disorders. Orthopedic surgeons will complete a five-year residency. They are taught to treat all aspects of bone care from traumatic fractures, tumors, degenerative arthritis, and sports-related injuries. They may specialize in joint replacement surgeries including knee, hip, and shoulder replacements. Arthroscopic procedures (endoscopic procedures involving the joints) are commonly done in the knee, shoulder, and more recently the hip. The arthroscopic approach can repair torn ligaments and fix tears in the lining of the joints (debridements). Other orthopedic surgeons may choose to do a one- to two-year fellowship and further specialize in tumor resection, trauma care, or spine surgeries.

Fracture care also remains a keystone of orthopedic care. They routinely perform surgeries to address fractures that include fractures that are not lined up, known as displaced fractures. The care of a displaced fracture may include placing the pieces in alignment, known as reduction or utilizing hardware (screws and plates) to get the bone pieces or fragments to align together. Treatment for a nondisplaced fracture may involve placing a cast on the injured extremity. The goal is to reduce movement at the fracture site to promote healing of the bone.

Medical Imaging

Radiologist

Radiologists are specialists who interpret diagnostic imaging studies. Radiologists will complete a four-year residency. They specialize in reading imaging studies. They are experts at reading CT scans, magnetic resonance imaging (MRI), radiographs (X-rays), and ultrasound studies. They may choose to do an interventional fellowship of one to two years and will gain the additional skills of being able to use CT or X-rays to place catheters or to perform interventions to treat problems.

CLINICAL PEARL

Board certification (BC) is the gold standard among physicians. This refers to the fact that the physician has completed a residency training program in his or her specialty as well as successfully passed an examination. This certification assures the patient of a certain level of standing. Board eligible (BE) denotes that the physician has completed the training but has not taken the test yet. Consumers should pursue physicians who are BC or BE whenever possible.

Chapter 3

Inpatient versus Outpatient Medicine

The terms "inpatient" and "outpatient" are very basic ones to understand. They simply refer to the location of care that is provided to a patient. *Inpatient care* is care administered to a patient admitted to a hospital, mental/behavioral health unit, nursing home, extended care facility, or other medical facility and who stays overnight or greater than 24 hours in such a facility. *Outpatient care* is the term reserved for a patient who is not hospitalized overnight but who visits a hospital, clinic, office for a check-up, or a facility for diagnosis or treatment.

Factors Impacting Delivery

Historically health care, including treatments and surgeries, were done in a hospital environment as inpatient medicine. However, there has been a significant increase and emphasis on outpatient services over the past twenty years. Trying to contain escalating costs has been the main factor in transitioning from an inpatient medical focus to the outpatient setting.

The creation of Medicare in 1966 expanded the number of insured Americans, thereby increasing the use of services and costs. With more covered lives comes higher costs. Technology also plays a significant role, and new technologies are associated with greater costs. Previous examples of some technologies include transplant surgeries, cardiac surgeries, and orthopedic joint replacements, all of which have become more common over the decade of the eighties and nineties.

Historically, hospitals were reimbursed retrospectively, meaning if the patient was in the hospital longer and had higher costs, the hospital was reimbursed more by Medicare. This system did little to contain the costs of inpatient care. The government, more specifically Medicare and insurers, have responded to the increase in medical costs. One such response is the prospective payment system, instituted on October 1, 1983.[1]

The prospective payment system will pay hospitals a predetermined fixed amount for care administered to a Medicare patient according to his or her particular diagnosis-related group (DRG). In other words, insurance companies will pay a fixed amount to the hospital for taking care of a patient with pneumonia, regardless of how many days the patient stays in the hospital and the associated costs. Each admitting diagnosis has a DRG associated with it. The bottom line is the hospital can make more money if the patient has a shorter length of stay and utilizes less resources (imaging studies, tests, and labs) during their stay in the hospital. However, to discourage premature discharges and inadequate care, the hospital can be fined and lose their Medicare payment if the patient is readmitted to the hospital within 30 days. The operating margins under the prospective payment system for inpatient hospital care are thin. This risk and low-profit margin have lead the shift toward outpatient treatment centers.

These centers are commonly known as an ambulatory care centers. *Ambulatory* indicates walking and being consistent with a certain degree of health. *Care* is synonymous with treatment, while *center* is suggestive of a setting of excellence incorporating advanced technologies.

Outpatient services are more cost effective than inpatient hospitals. The associated cost is less than in a hospital setting, as outpatient service centers do not require an overnight stay. In addition, outpatient service centers usually specialize in one type of treatment or procedure. By specializing in a certain procedure day after day, this repetitive exposure will give the staff a lot of experience that is focused on the procedure the patient needs. Staff are better suited to deal with any complications if they perform thousands of procedures per year, versus the staff at a center who may only perform a few a week. Specialization should also allow the center to acquire the most advanced equipment and perform the latest techniques, which are felt to produce improved outcomes and patient satisfaction.

Another patient convenience associated with outpatient services is that all care is provided in one place. All of the care that one needs before, during, and after his or her procedure, surgery, or test may be conveniently provided under one roof. Given the increase in ambulatory care centers over the past two decades, there is typically a facility that is geographically close and convenient to receive care.

Competition

Outpatient centers are profitable. Hospitals have little margin regarding inpatient care, while outpatient centers receive nice reimbursements for the care provided. Outpatient centers' operating costs tend to be lower with less variation due to the repetitive nature of the procedures being performed. The potential for profits has led to the proliferation of many ambulatory care centers. These centers may be owned by a hospital, health care plan, or privately by a medical group.

What factors are involved when choosing an ambulatory care center? Most patients will feel more comfortable in the care of a particular physician rather than a certain center. However, the likely determining factor in choosing a center will also depend on one's insurance plan. Consumers will likely choose a center designated as a preferred center or participating facility with their insurance plan.

Outpatient Care Centers

Outpatient or ambulatory care centers can provide a distinct number of services to patients (see table 3.1). The list of procedures and surgeries that can be performed at a surgical center is extensive. The APG ambulatory surgery procedure list is approximately 75 pages long. These surgeries may include but are in no means are limited to partial breast mastectomy, arthroscopic procedures of various joints, repair of nasal septum, and artery bypass grafting. It is more likely a surgery can be done at an ambulatory care center than not. Still, some surgeries are done in the hospital and require an overnight stay including joint replacements, surgery involving major organs, and the majority of spinal procedures.

TABLE 3.1   TYPES OF AMBULATORY CARE CENTERS

Surgery centers	Lab centers
Imaging centers	Gastrointestinal centers
Cardiac catherization centers	Durable medical equipment centers
Mental or behavioral health centers	Physical therapy centers
Substance abuse centers	Chemotherapy and radiation therapy centers

Imaging centers are another type of an ambulatory care center. These centers specialize in imaging of the body both for diagnosis and treatment. These centers will typically be anchored by magnetic resonance imaging (MRI). Studies to evaluate body structures by use of an MRI can confirm a patient's diagnosis and assist in directing treatments. In addition, some centers offer radiographic-guided therapeutic procedures. Examples may include using imaging to place stents in obstructed structures or performing vertebroplasties (using cement at the site of a spinal compression fracture to provide stability and reduce pain).

Laboratory centers specialize in drawing and processing lab specimens and tests. The blood can be drawn and the results run on the sample taken. Such centers will have experienced phlebotomists, individuals who draw blood samples on patients. These centers can be very convenient for patients to have blood work done rather than done in a hospital.

Gastrointestinal centers, which may provide screening or other services such as colonoscopy and endoscopy, are also becoming more common. These centers will specialize in procedures to evaluate the upper gastrointestinal tract (endoscopy) or the lower gastrointestinal tract and rectum (colonoscopy). Such centers will perform thousands of these studies in a year and will become very proficient in this procedure.

In addition, physical therapy centers are another example of an ambulatory care center. Therapy centers will be staffed by a number of physical therapists. Such centers, given the number of physical therapists on site, will have a greater likelihood of having certain therapists subspecialize. These subspecializations may better address the diagnosis of back pain, lymphedema (swelling of an extremity), stroke, and spinal cord injury.

Ambulatory care centers continue to serve as convenient sites to provide and administer medical care and treatments for patients and likely will continue to play a significant role in health care delivery in the future.

Inpatient Care

While there has been a dramatic shift in the number of outpatient versus inpatient admissions over the past two decades, there is still a need for inpatient care. One is typically admitted to the hospital when more intensive monitoring or specialized care is required.

Admission to a Hospital

Patients are admitted to a hospital by one of three ways: after evaluation in the emergency room (ER), direct admission from a physician's office or outpatient clinic, or via transfer from another hospital or medical facility. See Table 3.2.

TABLE 3.2   ADMISSION TO A HOSPITAL

After evaluation in the Emergency Room (ER)
Direct admission from a physician's office or outpatient clinic
Transfer from another hospital or medical facility

For admission into the hospital, certain criteria need to be met. These criteria may include failure to respond to outpatient treatment with worsening of the patient's clinical condition. Another reason for admission is that the current treatment plan will continue to be modified and such changes to the treatment program are best done in an inpatient hospital setting. The most common reason for an inpatient admission is an abrupt change in medical status including but not limited to chest pain, mental status changes, and new onset of neurologic deficits. Additionally, the patient may be admitted to the hospital after a 23-hour period of observation in the emergency room, where his or her condition has not and is not expected to improve.

Physician Orders

Patients who are admitted to a hospital are usually admitted under the care or service of a physician or physician group. It is important for consumers to understand the role of the *admitting* or *attending* physician. The admitting physician is responsible for supervising and ordering care for the patient. What orders are typically written by the admitting or attending physician? The attending physician will order every aspect of the patient's care.

The initial order is the admit order; the physician will provide this order to initiate admission to the hospital and to specify the level of care at the hospital. The physician will also be responsible for the discharge order, dismissing one from the hospital. The level of care provided to the patient can range from an intensive care unit, regular floor, operating room, or behavioral health unit. The specific unit is based on the medical needs and status of the patient.

Any pertinent precautions will also be outlined by the attending physician; these may include fall risks, seizure precautions, or non-weight-bearing to any extremity recovering from a fracture. Vital signs performed by the nursing staff, which include obtaining the patient's temperature, heart rate, breathing or respiration rate, and blood pressure, will be ordered at specific frequencies. These will be more frequent for unstable or critical patients and less frequent for more medically stable patients. It is a positive sign when the frequency of monitoring a patient's vital signs is reduced, as it typically signifies improvement in his or her medical condition. The patient's activity will also be addressed by the attending physician as he or she may choose bed rest, out of bed (OOB) with supervision, or ad lib (as able). Patients unable to drink enough fluid may require intravenous supplementation with an IV.

The patient's diet will also be ordered by the physician and may include low sodium for patients with high blood pressure, cardiac diet low in saturated fats for patients with cardiac concerns, or a pureed diet with thickened liquids for patients following a stroke, which has affected the patient's ability to safely swallow. Any allergies will also need to be noted in the orders to prevent patients from receiving a medication that could cause a significant reaction or anaphylactic (life-threatening) reaction. Likewise, any medications that the patient should or will need to be taking will be outlined in the orders. Consults for physicians in different specialties may also be ordered for their input to help with the care of the patient. Any lab or diagnostic tests, including X-rays, CT scans, EKGs, or MRIs, will also be ordered by the attending physician.

It is important to remember to check with the nursing staff to know of any activity precautions or dietary concerns that may be ordered for a family member during his or her stay in the hospital. Knowing any limitations can help prevent complications that may arise.

CLINICAL PEARL

Medicare may reimburse the physician at different rates for the same services based on the location of the service. When comparing three different patient settings, the physician's office, hospital outpatient department, and an ambulatory surgery center, the amount the physician was paid in 2013 for performing an epidural injection was $211.96 in a physician's office, $407.28 in an ambulatory surgery center, and $655.62 in a hospital outpatient department. The different reimbursement rates can significantly influence the location of care.[2]

Endnotes

1. Stuart Guterman and Allen Dobson, "Impact of the Medicare Prospective Payment System for Hospitals," *Health Care Financing Review* 7, no. 3 (1986): 97–114.
2. Laxmaiah Manchikanti, Ramsin Benyamin, Frank J. E. Falco, and Joshua A. Hirsch, "Recommendations of the Medicare Payment Advisory Commission (MEDPAC) on the Health Care Delivery System: The impact on Interventional Pain Management in 2014 and Beyond," *Pain Physician* 16, no. 5 (2013): 419–40.

Chapter 4

Selecting and Navigating Physicians' Offices

Recently a patient joked with me that he does not want to be treated by a doctor, but rather the doctor's doctor. I both appreciated and understood his humor. This chapter serves to inform the consumer of the important factors to consider when selecting a physician and provides strategies for patients to get the most of their visit. The chapter presents a doctor's guide on finding a doctor.

Office Visits

The majority of health care administered in the United States is not in a hospital, but at an outpatient office visit. According to the Centers for Disease Control and Prevention (CDC) and the 2015 National Ambulatory Medical Care Survey, there were 990.8 million outpatient or office visits. The survey also notes that the average number of visits per person per year was 3.13. The majority of visits (51%) were to a primary care physician. The most commonly diagnosed condition during these visits is arthritis and its related complications.[1]

Options

Consumers have three main categories of doctors to choose from: a physician in academic practice, a physician who is employed by a healthcare system, and a physician who is in private practice. The differences are summarized in table 4.1.

TABLE 4.1   DIFFERENT PHYSICIAN OPTIONS

Type	Pros	Cons
Academic	Complete visits	Long visits with multiple learners
Employed	Associated with a health system	Pressures to perform
Private Practice	Efficient and convenient visits	Financial incentives to see and do more

An academic physician, also known as an attending physician, works for a medical school and treats patients but also educates physicians in training including medical students, interns, residents, and fellows. These physicians are very knowledgeable in terms of the latest treatments and evidence-based medicine. Another advantage that the medical school may offer is a clinical trial or novel treatment for patients not available in other settings. When patients schedule an appointment with an academic physician, they may first be evaluated by a physician in training, a resident or a student. The physician in training will then present the patient's history and examination findings to the attending physician. The attending physician will likely confirm important parts of his or her history and may repeat certain portions of the physical examination. While a visit to an academic physician may take a longer amount of time, the visit will be complete and comprehensive.

The *employed* physician is employed by a healthcare organization. The doctor is usually associated with other physicians and specialists in the health care network or organization. Some healthcare systems may be associated with resident training programs, but not typically medical students. The employed physician visit has the advantage of having accessibility to other providers and specialists within in the healthcare system. This can lead to prompt evaluations and treatments. In today's economic environment, the employed physician is under pressure to see a certain number of patients per week and likely has a base salary tied to an incentive bonus, based on production for the healthcare system. The number of employed physicians has steadily increased over the past decade, while the number of private practice physicians has declined.

Choosing a physician in private practice is another option. Private practice physicians may be affiliated with a hospital but are not employed by the hospital. Their practice is based on providing good and efficient care to patients. They may offer extended office hours with convenient accessibility including parking. They are usually not associated with residents or other physicians in training. A private practice physician has a financial incentive to see patients and perform procedures or surgeries; for this reason, visits tend to be efficient and these physicians may be more likely to recommend a procedure.

Charges

A patient may be billed differently, dependent on the physician type he or she sees. The academic physician will submit a bill for professional charges. This includes any procedures that the physician performs in the academic medical center. The patient may also receive a facility fee. This is the cost associated with having a procedure done at that particular facility. An employed physician will bill for a professional component and the healthcare system may submit an additional facility fee charge. A private practice physician will submit a single global fee that includes the professional component and facility usage of the bill.

Establishing Care

Choosing the right physician is very important. Unfortunately, your choice may be limited. Your insurance plan may list "in-network" physicians or health care providers, limiting your choice from a financial perspective. You may choose a healthcare provider out of network, but the costs you incur may only be partially or not at all covered by your plan. Therefore, most consumers will start their search with their in-network care providers.

The best way to know which providers are "in network" is to call your insurance plan or obtain your in-network list from the insurance website. Use your insurer's directory or search on its website for doctors in your network.

Most providers will accept Medicare. Finding a physician who accepts Medicaid may be more challenging, particularly with private care providers. It is best to confirm that your insurance product is accepted at your prospective physician's office before initiating any type of evaluation or care.

Board Certification

Board certification is considered the gold standard within the medical field. Being certified through the American Board of Medical Specialties (ABMS) means a doctor has earned a medical degree from a qualified medical school, completed three to seven years of accredited residency training, is licensed by a state medical board, and has passed one or more exams administered by the ABMS. To maintain the certification, the doctor also participates in a continuing education program. Board eligible means that the physician has completed all components of the process but has not taken and passed the examination. Board eligible is a common status for physicians who have very recently completed a residency program and who have not yet taken their examination. The examinations are usually offered once a year. Consumers should be aware of their prospective physician's board status.

Websites

The internet has websites available with additional information on physicians for consumers. These sites can be helpful, but some sites and content should be approached with caution. There are sites that list the doctor's education, training, and areas of expertise. This is valuable objective information. In addition, any sanctions, malpractice claims, and insurance plans accepted by the physician may also be listed. Subjective information including patient satisfaction and ratings may also appear.

Healthgrades.com is a useful site that includes information on education, affiliated hospitals (and ratings on the hospital itself), sanctions, malpractice claims and board actions, office locations, and insurance plans. The site will also include additional information on patient satisfaction and wait times. The link is www.healthgrades.com.

Another site for consumers is Vitals.com. This site can assist in finding doctors by their specialty, the patient's condition, and insurance plan. The site also includes information regarding the physician's awards, expertise, hospital affiliations, insurance plans, and patient ratings. There is also a patient-comment section. The link is www.vitals.com.

The U.S. News & World Report site does not provide ratings of doctors, but it can be a very helpful site when choosing a physician. The site contains information on the physician's education, training, years in practice, hospital affiliations, certification, licensure, insurance plans, publications, and awards. The link for the site is health.usnews.com/doctors.

Online Resources

Caution should be exercised for the subjective information found on the sites. There is no guarantee the information is accurate. Anyone can access and submit a physician rating online. There is currently no way to validate the patient comments or rating sections on the sites. A very unhappy patient or a competing provider can leave factitious comments or low ratings to adversely affect a physician. Conversely, the physician or his or her staff can submit very positive comments in an effort to improve patient recruitment. The internal hospital ratings of providers avoid this potential problem by offering surveys only to treated patients and is usually then compiled by a private third-party company.

While it is very important to review and consider a prospective physician's education, training, and certifications, less emphasis should be placed on the subjective measures.

Appointment Scheduling

Your time to see a physician is typically scheduled, meaning you cannot simply show up to be seen. Unfortunately, it is not uncommon to wait in the office well beyond your scheduled appointment time. Some waits can be longer than 90 minutes, most are less than 20 minutes. Why the delay in being seen later than your scheduled appointment? One reason is the complexity of the patient's problem(s). Patients may indicate a relatively simple problem when the appointment is made, but additional time may be needed during the appointment to better understand the problem.

Also, commonly patients will have more than one problem they wish to have addressed at their appointment. Physicians may address more than one issue during the scheduled appointment, but this is the exception rather than the norm. Most physicians will address only one problem per visit. Addressing multiple issues requires extra time and the extra time can certainly delay the physician's schedule as the day goes on.

Another reason for increased wait times are due to late-arriving patients. If the ten o'clock patient arrives seven minutes late, then all subsequent patients will likely be delayed seven minutes. The last and most recent factor is the advent of the electronic medical record. This system adds additional time per patient to satisfy the multiple regulations that are required in terms of the process of the patient.

Appointment

When arriving to the office, you will notify the staff of your presence and appointment. The staff are not permitted to identify you by your last name because of the Health Insurance Portability and Accountability Act of 1996 (HIPAA), **thus the staff will call** you by your first name. Once you are called the nursing staff will take you to an examination room and obtain vital signs. These are standard measurements of temperature, heart rate, breathing rate, and blood pressure. Most offices will also obtain height and weight measurements.

A medical intake form may have been sent prior to your appointment or can be filled out in the office while you are waiting for your physician or care provider to enter the room. The medical intake form may also be done verbally, providing information to the nursing staff electronically into your medical record. The staff will also ask you the reason for your visit; this is known as the "chief complaint." Certain care providers may stick to the one-visit-one-problem approach. They will also review your past medical history. It is best to bring in any previous medical records if you are unsure or cannot recall them.

Allergies to medications will also be reviewed. It is important to note the distinction between an *allergy* and a *sensitivity*. A true allergy is a reaction, occasionally life threatening to a medication. It can involve swelling of the lips, tongue, or throat or the development of an itchy rash. Sensitivities to drugs are not severe reactions and may include nausea, diarrhea, sedation, and headache. These sensitivities result from use of the medicine but are not life threatening.

Any current medications that the patient is taking must also be reviewed. It is best to actually bring in the medication bottles to reference exactly what you are taking. Telling the nurse or physician you are taking a small pink pill does not help. Many medications look alike and one generic producer may produce a tablet or capsule of a different color or shape than another manufacturer of the same medication.

You will also want to provide an accurate social history. The social history entails occupational or vocational review as well discussing alcohol or tobacco use. Family history may also be helpful in having knowledge of certain diseases that run in the family. Knowing the health history of one's parents and siblings can be very beneficial. Lastly, you may be asked to fill out a review of systems form. This will ask a number of questions related to the health or medical issues of the different systems of the body and may include the following: cardiac, pulmonary, neurologic, and orthopedic.

Then the physician, nurse practitioner, physician's assistant (PA), or another care provider will enter the room. It is important to know that your scheduled appointment will likely be between 20–45 minutes for a new patient visit and between 10–20 minutes for a follow-up visit. To get the most out of your visit it is best to be clear and concise with your description of the problem. For example when asked how long have you had the pain, you should respond with a time duration answer; it is not the time to get into overly descriptive details of the day (i.e., weather), what you were wearing the day the pain started or how your normal routine was disrupted and the consequences that occurred. The correct answer takes seconds, whereas the less appropriate convoluted approach takes minutes. The latter also doesn't actually answer the original question and squanders the patient of valuable time. If the physician or care provider feels additional details are helpful, he or she will ask you to elaborate further.

Physical Examination

The hallmark of any office visit is the physical examination. These have been performed by doctors for over two thousand years. The healthcare provider will perform a physical examination. Depending on the problem, the examination may be comprehensive or focused. Comprehensive examinations will include examinations of multiple parts (organs) of the body, which may help in making a correct diagnosis. The focused examination will only examine areas of the body that are related to the chief complaint.

Expectations

Following a medical office visit, you should be provided with the following: diagnosis (cause of your disease, problem or illness), answers to any questions you had, and a plan. Sometimes the diagnosis is not obvious and will require additional testing; in these cases a differential diagnosis (a number of possible explanations) should be discussed and reviewed. You, as a patient, are paying for the services of the physician and should ask any questions you have in terms of the diagnosis, treatment plan, and follow-up care. Lastly, all visits should end with a plan or recommendation. The plan may include medications, therapies, or additional testing. What happens when your expectations are not met? You the consumer are paying for your medical evaluation as well as the attention and time of the medical professional to provide an appropriate and acceptable treatment plan. Consumers should feel empowered to have any of their questions regarding alternate treatments addressed and not dismissed and feel that their needs have been met.

Results

One chooses a physician to manage his or her medical conditions and maximize his or her outcomes. Most businesses are results driven. If you went to a restaurant and did not enjoy the meal, would you go back to the same restaurant? The same thinking should apply with your healthcare provider. It is important to ask yourself, am I getting better? If the answer is no, then you may wish to obtain a second opinion from another physician. It is concerning if your physician or healthcare provider is offended by letting him or her know you are planning to seek a second opinion. In cases where elective surgery is recommended (not life-threatening conditions or urgent surgery), seeking a second opinion should be sought.

CLINICAL PEARL

Best appointment times: There are certain appointment times where the wait time in the office can be significantly reduced. The first appointment of the day and the first appointment after lunch are prime spots to schedule in order to minimize your wait time. The first patient has the advantage of not following any patient, so it is very likely the provider will start on time. The wait times typically increase as the day goes on. This delay can reset after the lunch break and build again as the day progresses.

Resources

Healthgrades: Website that allows consumers to identify a physician by specialty or location, site also provides education, experience, certification, and patient feedback: http://www.healthgrades.com/

Vitals: Webpage that allows consumers to search a location for a physician, this site also provides information on the physician's address, education, reviews, and participating insurance plans: http://www.vitals.com/

U.S. News & World Report: Link for physician information website that provides contact information, insurance, education, and experiences for the physician: http://health.usnews.com/doctors

Endnote

1. "Ambulatory Health Care Data," *National Center for Health Statistics.* 2015, https://www.cdc.gov/nchs/ahcd/index.htm.

Chapter 5

Testing and Diagnoses

I f you have ever watched a medical drama on television
or via other media, the doctor is usually calling out
orders to be done for the patient. The physician may be
ordering a CBC or lytes and wanting them stat (stat means
as fast as possible in medicine). This chapter will address
what tests are typically done, why they are ordered, and
how they help in providing care for the patient.

Diagnosis

"Diagnosis" is the medical term used to define the determining cause of one's medical symptoms. It involves the
process of concluding the underlying cause of the patient's
problems. The diagnosis is based on the patient's history,
examination, and review of laboratory data. It is commonly
taught in medical school that the history and physical examination should provide the correct diagnosis about 75%
of the time. Therefore, diagnostic tests can be helpful to
confirm the diagnosis. Tests can also follow the clinical

status of the disease process or help narrow the diagnosis if it is uncertain or unknown.

Diagnostic tests are medical procedures that can include laboratory tests, imaging tests and other specialized tests. Laboratory tests are medical procedures that involve testing samples of blood, urine, tissues, or substances in the body. Imaging tests help to evaluate the anatomy of the body. Specialized tests are used to evaluate the functioning or physiology of the body and can include electrocardiograms (EKG), sleep studies, pulmonary function tests, and electroencephalogram (EEG) procedures.

Complete Blood Count

Common blood tests involve analysis of blood cells, electrolytes, and the function of certain organs. The complete blood count (CBC) test looks at the population of blood cells in the body. Blood cells are produced by the bone marrow. Marrow is found in the middle or hollow portion of the long bones of our body. The marrow produces three main lines of cells: white cells, red cells, and platelets.

The three lines of cells perform different functions for the body. The white blood cells (WBC), also known as *leukocytes*, form the basis for our immune system. Our immune system is paramount in fighting infections. The infections that are caused by foreign invaders may include bacteria, viruses, or fungus, all of which can cause illness. The red blood cells (RBC), also known as *erythrocytes*, function to carry oxygen to the various organs of the body. Oxygen is the fuel for sustained cell functions. Without oxygen the cells will not be able to function and will die. The *platelets* are the last main component of the blood. They function to prevent and stop bleeding by clumping together to form clots.

The CBC is ordered to evaluate the status of the three main cell lines. The blood test can give information about potential problems. There are normal ranges and parameters for each of the different cell lines. If the WBCs or leukocytes are elevated, this may suggest an infection or leukemia. The WBCs can continue to be monitored to ensure the treatments are adequately addressing the problem. Low WBCs can be caused by viral infections, seen with chemotherapy, a toxic reaction, or a problem with the bone marrow that produces the cells.

The WBCs are able to be differentiated further into 5 subtypes, neutrophils eosinophils, basophils, monocytes, and lymphocytes, based on their specific function. When the CBC is ordered the ordering physician may request a manual differential. This entails having someone review the blood sample under a microscope and analyzing (counting) the different subtypes of WBCs.

Neutrophils focus on fighting infections caused by bacteria and fungus. Lymphocytes can be further differentiated into T and B cells. T cells aid in recognizing infections and activate other immune cells while B cells produce antibodies, which target and destroy invading germs. Monocytes are cells that may transform into macrophages. These cells can then engulf and eliminate infectious organisms, particularly bacteria. Eosinophils are important in fighting parasitic infections and are also involved with allergic responses. Lastly, basophils are also important mediators in the allergy cascade.

The RBCs or erythrocytes provide information about the oxygen-carrying capacity in one's blood. The lab will describe the patient's RBC capacity in terms of *hematocrit* and *hemoglobin*. Hematocrit is the volume of red blood cells in your body and it specifically measures the ratio of RBCs in your blood. Hemoglobin is the iron containing protein molecule in red blood cells that carries oxygen. Low RBC counts are known as anemia. Anemias can be caused by blood loss (bleeding) or lack of production by the marrow. Inadequate iron may be a cause of a production problem. RBCs are monitored to assess the patient's response to treatment.

Platelets are also measured. Low platelet counts are known as *thrombocytopenia* and are normally caused by either a lack of production or an increase in destruction. Potential causes of low production thrombocytopenia include viruses, leukemias, and chemotherapy. Increased destruction causes are seen with pregnancy and autoimmune diseases.

Electrolytes

Electrolytes are electrically charged ions that regulate our nerve and muscle function and play a role in our body's pH. They exert control over ion channels in the nerves and muscles by generating electricity, contracting muscles, and affecting fluid concentrations within the body. The major electrolytes found within the body include sodium, potassium, calcium, magnesium, phosphate, and chloride. The concentration of electrolytes in the body is dependent on intake (diet) because they cannot be produced by the body. Once in the body, they are regulated by *hormones*. The hormones managing electrolyte concentrations are mainly produced by the kidneys and the adrenal glands. Sensors are located within the kidneys, which monitor the specific concentrations of the electrolytes. The kidneys determine when to filter (keep) and when to excrete (get rid of) the various electrolytes.

Because the electrolytes play an important role in nerve and muscle activities, an imbalance of electrolytes can cause significant problems. The lab test that is ordered to evaluate the electrolytes involves taking a small sample of blood. It is commonly referred to as the basic metabolic panel (BMP) or the chem 8 and "lytes" in the movies or on television/media shows.

The electrolytes, sodium, potassium, chloride, carbon dioxide (bicarbonate), and calcium account for five tests. Glucose, blood urea nitrogen, and creatinine make up the remaining three components. Together, they will help to provide the necessary concentrations of the electrolytes in the body. Knowing the concentration can also provide important information as to the status of the kidneys and respiratory system.

Blood Glucose

Glucose is a sugar. Its concentrations are regulated by hormones produced by the pancreas. The hormone that *lowers* the blood glucose level is *insulin*. The hormone that *raises* the blood glucose level is *glucagon*. The levels of glucose are tested to determine if one has diabetes mellitus, which would be suggested with an elevated (high) fasting (before meals) blood glucose level. The level of glucose is expected to rise after eating a meal. In response, the body releases insulin to lower the level of glucose in the blood stream. With diabetes, the body is unable to produce enough insulin or the body has developed a degree of resistance to the insulin and the blood glucose levels remain high. Elevated blood glucose levels over time can lead to destruction of nerves and injury to very small blood vessels. These injuries can lead to blindness; loss of sensation in the feet, hands, and legs; and kidney damage. Medications can help to improve blood glucose levels. Patients with diabetes, known as diabetics, must monitor their blood glucose levels regularly to ensure the medication responses are adequate and the degree of damage is minimized.

Liver Function Tests

The blood test that specifically evaluates the components of enzymes and proteins that are associated with proper functioning of the liver are known as liver function tests (LFTs). The liver is the largest internal organ of the body (second overall to the skin). The liver serves many functions within the body. The liver function tests will look at each of the specific functions of the liver.

The liver is responsible for detoxification. It contains a number of enzymes that are responsible for converting drugs, alcohol, and toxins into harmless products that the body will eliminate with bile in intestines or excrete via the kidneys. Nutrients are also processed in the liver after they are digested. The liver will also produce *bile*, which is stored in the gall bladder and used to help break down fats and remove waste from the body. The liver also produces proteins necessary for blood clotting. The liver is also important for storage of fat-soluble vitamins as well as converting glucose into glycogen for storage.

Kidney Function tests

Kidney function tests are blood tests that are ordered to evaluate the functional status of the kidneys. These paired organs are located in the retro (behind) peritoneal (abdominal cavity) region. The kidneys are responsible for filtering and excreting waste products from the blood. They also assist in maintaining electrolyte balance and red blood cell production.

The specific tests of interest are the blood urea nitrogen (BUN), creatinine (Cr), and the glomerular filtration rate (GFR). When the kidneys become impaired they are not able to actively secrete urea and creatinine out of the body and their levels become elevated. The GFR measures the ability of the kidney to filter; a normal level is greater than 60. A level lower than 60 but greater than 15 indicates kidney or renal impairment. Renal failure is a level that is lower than 15. The kidney function tests can identify a problem associated with the kidneys but does not specifically diagnose the problem. Kidney disease can be caused by the following: a problem with the blood flow before it enters the kidney (pre-renal), problems of the kidney itself (renal), or an issue in the ureters or bladder (post-renal). Additional testing may be needed to further locate the exact cause.

Imaging Tests

Radiograph is a photographic image produced by the action of an electromagnetic wave of high energy and known more commonly as an X-ray. To obtain an X-ray the patient is positioned between the X-ray source and a detector (film), and then the beam of energy will pass through the body. When the X-ray passes through the different parts of the body, each part will absorb the X-rays in different amounts. The density of the tissue will determine how much radiation is absorbed. Bones, which are dense and made of calcium, will absorb more of the X-rays than softer tissues, which include organs, muscles, and fat. The denser structures will appear white and softer structures will range from more than fifty shades of gray to black.

X-rays are used commonly in patients to evaluate the status of a bone and the condition of the lungs. When evaluating the status of a bone or bones, the X-ray can reveal if a bone is broken or fractured. It can determine if the fracture is compound (multiple pieces) or displaced (edges of the fractures are not close to each other). Knowing this information helps to guide appropriate treatment. The X-rays can also show if the fracture and bone is healing appropriately. New bone growth at a fracture site is known as *callus*, and serial radiographs can be taken to show the various stages of healing and callus formation.

Radiographs can also assist in gaining information about various diseases involving the lung. Radiograph films can show lung changes that occur with chronic obstructive pulmonary disease (COPD); they may also show the presence of a lung tumor or cancer. In addition, X-rays may reveal a pneumonia (infection of the lung) as well as the presence of heart congestion and subsequent fluid build-up in the lungs. Lastly, the chest X-ray can reveal the presence of a pneumothorax (collapsed lung), which is a concern following trauma to the chest.

Computerized Tomography (CT) Scan

A computerized tomography (CT) scan, also known as a CAT scan, uses radiation to obtain a more detailed view of the body than regular radiographs. It was invented by an engineer, Godfrey Hounsfield, who was awarded the Nobel Prize in medicine and was promoted by a neuroradiologist, Dr. James Ambrose, who demonstrated its wide clinical significance.[1] While the radiograph sends out a single X-ray; the CAT scan sends out several beams from different angles. The different images are then processed by a computer to create axial (cross-sectional) images of the body. These images allow for greater detail from within the body to be analyzed. The images are typically interpreted by a radiologist. The CAT scan uses radiation to obtain the images.

The CAT scanner invented by Hounsfield was originally designed to take pictures of the brain. It has been advanced and is now used to take images throughout the body. Advantages of the CAT scan include the speed in obtaining the images and the ability to see views of structures within the body. It is for this reason that the CAT scan is used in the initial evaluation of stroke patients who arrive at the hospital. The CAT scan can show if the suspected stroke is caused by a bleed or is related to ischemia (lack of blood flow). Knowing this can direct the initial treatment of the stoke patient and lead to an improved outcome.

CAT scan imaging can be done preoperatively to evaluate a mass or tumor that can assist the surgeon in removal, as well as guide an interventional radiologist in obtaining a biopsy of an organ or tissue sample. The CAT scan is particularly useful for evaluating bone and detecting the presence of a nondisplaced fracture, which may not show on a standard X-ray. The scans can also be used to follow an aortic abdominal aneurysm for assessing enlargements. CAT scans are also used by radiation oncologists to precisely pinpoint the tumor for treatment with a beam of radiation.

Bone Scan

A bone scan is a nuclear imaging test that helps diagnose and track several types of bone problems. The testing procedure involves injecting a small amount of radioactive dye typically into a vein of the arm. Following injection of the dye, X-ray pictures of the body are then taken. The X-rays can be of the entire body or a specific area of concern. Depending on the reason for of the test, additional X-rays may be taken again after a period of between two and four hours. The uptake of the dye will be increased in "hot spots." Hot spots or areas of concern include infections, fractures (not apparent on regular X-rays), and metastatic cancers of the bone and will be noted with an increase update of dye into these areas.

The test is ordered to help diagnose a bone tumor or cancer, an infection of bone, a fracture, Paget's disease (metabolic bone disorder), or an unexplained cause of bone pain.

Ultrasound

Diagnostic ultrasound, also called *sonography*, is an imaging method that uses high-frequency sound waves to produce images of structures within the body. The procedure uses a transducer, which is placed on skin that has been treated with ultrasound gel. The transducer produces high frequency sound waves that enter the body and are sent back to the transducer, which then relays the information to a computer for analysis of the information and creation of an image. The information is helpful for diagnosing and treating a variety of diseases as well as evaluating a fetus for growth or structural problems. The test does not use radiation. The test is used frequently to evaluate blood flow in vessels, assess the presence of a blood clot, or to diagnose gall bladder disease. Diagnostic ultrasound is typically noninvasive, but special transducers exist that can be inserted into the esophagus to get better imaging of the heart, into a male's rectum to get images of the prostate, and also into a women's vagina to better evaluate the uterus and ovaries.

Presently, ultrasound is being used for anatomical identification of body structures such as tendons, muscles, joints, vessels, and internal organs. Physicians may use the ultrasound to guide injections into these specific areas and structures.

Magnetic Resonance Imaging

Magnetic resonance imaging (MRI) is a test that uses a magnetic field and radio waves. The information is processed by a computer, which then produces very detailed images of structures inside the body. Since the test uses a magnetic field, patients with an implanted pacemaker and other metal devices may not be able to have an

MRI. Additionally, construction workers and welders may need to be screened before having an MRI to ensure that they do not have metal fragments in their eyes. MRI is a safe imaging alternative for pregnant woman as it does not utilize radiation.

For an MRI test, the area of the body being studied is placed inside a tube that contains a strong magnet. Patients who have claustrophobia or difficulty being in tight spaces may require sedation to have the procedure, which can take up to 90 minutes to complete. The MRI scan will obtain very detailed images of structures within the body. It can be especially helpful in viewing soft tissues including the brain and spinal column. The test can also be ordered with dye or contrast material, and this may be injected to provide even better detail. The contrast material may be injected into the shoulder joint to better show a labral tear of the soft tissues within the shoulder joint or be used for a spinal MRI to help differentiate scar tissue from a recurrent disc herniation.

The disadvantages of the test are the associated costs, and most need to be approved by the patient's insurance company. The various imaging studies are summarized in table 5.1.

TABLE 5.1   COMPARISON OF DIAGNOSTIC IMAGING TECHNIQUES

Test	Positives	Negatives	Costs	Uses
X-rays	Quick, easy Screening tool	Not great detail	$	Assess for fracture Evaluation of lungs
CAT scan	Great for bone	Radiation	$$	Evaluation of stroke
Bone scan	Very sensitive for bony issues	Limited to bone problems	$$	Assessment of bone pain and infections
Ultra-sound	No radiation	Cannot assess deep structures	$	Fetal assessment Assess for blood clots
MRI	No radiation	Cannot have if implanted metal	$$$	Soft tissue, brain, and spine imaging

CLINICAL PEARL

CT scans expose the body to large amounts of radiation. How much? If you compare the amount of radiation the body is exposed to with a standard chest X-ray compared to a chest CAT scan it is approximately the equivalent of having 350 chest X-rays.[2] There are clear indications to have a CAT scan, such as in the case to evaluate stroke patients for the presence of a bleed and in other serious medical problems. The test should be ordered if it will likely change the treatment approach and affect outcome.

Resources

National Institute of Diabetes and Digestive and Kidney Diseases: Webpage outlines basics of kidney diseases and how to monitor/treat the various conditions: https://www.niddk.nih.gov/health-information/ health-communication-programs/nkdep/learn/causes-kidney-disease/ testing/understand-gfr/Pages/understand-gfr.aspx

National Institute of Biomedical Imaging and Bioengineering: NIH-sponsored site that goes into nice explanations and detail of what is involved with the various imaging studies: https://www.nibib.nih.gov/ science-education/science-topics/x-rays

Endnotes

1. Vladimir Petrik, Vinothini Apok, Juliet A. Britton, Ba Bell, and Marios Papadopoulos, "Godfrey Hounsfield and the Dawn of Computed Tomography," Neurosurgery 58, no. 4 (2006): 780–7.
2. Cynthia H., McCollough, Jerrold T. Bushberg, Joel Garland Fletcher, and Laurence J. Eckel, "Answers to Common Questions about the Use and Safety of CT scans," *Mayo Clinic Proceedings* 90, no. 10 (2015): 1380–92.

Chapter 6

Guide to Prescriptions

This chapter serves to give the consumer background information to the pharmaceutical industry and its influence on physicians. Additionally, drug development and classifications of the various medications will be reviewed. Lastly, the chapter will focus on strategies for finding the best price for medications.

Industry

The pharmaceutical industry develops, produces, and markets drugs: pharmaceuticals to treat diseases and ailments. The market is dominated by a few companies that produce and advertise the drugs. The companies are large and control a majority of the market. According to the World Health Organization (WHO), the 10 largest drugs companies control over one-third of this market, with several companies having sales of more than $10 billion a year and profit margins of about 30%. Six of the top ten companies are based in the United States and four in Europe.[1,2]

Development

Today medications in the United States undergo rigorous clinical trials and testing. Testing was implemented following the thalidomide tragedy in the 1960s. Thalidomide was a German-produced drug used to treat morning sickness during pregnancy. It was not extensively tested in pregnant animals, which was the standard of the time. Unfortunately, the medication was associated with disastrous side effects of the unborn fetuses. Children were born either without or severely deformed arms and legs. As a result of this tragedy the World Medical Association set standards for clinical research.

Pharmaceutical companies are now required to prove efficacy and safety of the drug in clinical trials before marketing them. This includes a four-step process, which is overseen by the Food and Drug Administration (FDA) in the United States. Phase 1 of testing includes drug tests in a small group of about twenty to one hundred healthy volunteers. Testing is done to determine the *safety* of the drug. If the drug is not safe and causes significant side effects or cannot be tolerated the testing will stop at this phase. If the drug is found to be safe for human consumption, further testing will proceed. According to the FDA, about 70% of drugs pass this initial phase of testing.

The second phase of testing will involve 100 to 500 volunteer patients in controlled trials. The purpose of the second phase is to determine *efficacy* (whether the medicine is effective) in treating the disease as well as looking at side effects. If found in controlled trials to be effective, drug testing moves to the next phase. The FDA estimates that 33% of medications will pass phase 2 testing and move to the third phase of testing.

During the third phase, one thousand to five thousand patients take the drug and are monitored to confirm effectiveness of the product and to identify *side effects*. This trial will have some of the volunteers take the new medication and others take a placebo (compound or intervention with no active drug effects, such as a sugar pill). This comparison will be done to compare the side effects of the medication with the placebo. The FDA estimates 25–30% of medications pass this phase.

The final phase is the fourth phase, and these trials are carried out once the drug has been approved by FDA during the post-market safety monitoring. In summary, for every one hundred drugs produced, seventy will make it to phase 2, 23 will make it to phase 3, and six medications will be approved by the FDA after a period of testing of ranging from two to seven years. Once the drug has been approved for use, the focus of the drug company then turns to marketing of the drug.

Research

Drug companies spend one-third of all sales revenue on marketing products—roughly twice what they spend on research and development. This emphasis on marketing their products has led some groups, including the World Health Organization (WHO), to express concerns. According to the WHO there is "an inherent conflict of interest between the legitimate business goals of manufacturers and the social, medical and economic needs of providers and the public to select and use drugs in the most rational way."[2]

This is particularly true where drugs companies are the main source of information as to which products are most effective. The industry expanded rapidly in the sixties, benefiting from new discoveries, and there were attempts to limit the financial links between drug companies and physicians. No legislation was enacted at that time. Without limits, the industry created and effectively used sales representatives to influence the medications physicians prescribe.

Marketing

The pharmaceutical industry has historically utilized sales representatives, also known as drug reps, to influence physicians' prescribing patterns. Their goal is to increase the sale of their assigned medications. The company will track how well the drug rep is doing based on sales of that drug in that particular region. One drug rep, Gwen Olsen, has written a book *Confessions of an Rx Drug Pusher*, detailing her 15 years as a pharmaceutical representative and her experiences.

Out of concern of the influence drug reps have on physician prescribing patterns, academic medical centers have restricted or limited the access of drug reps. The pharmaceutical industry strategized through another approach. The industry enlisted the assistance of physicians to inform other physicians of the products.

Pharmaceutical companies may sponsor a dinner, typically at a very nice restaurant, and employ a physician to lecture at the dinner. At these events a physician talks about the merits of a particular medication the company is sponsoring. In exchange, the physician who speaks will receive a *honoria* (payment) for the lecture. This approach has been proven to be very effective. "An internal study done by Merck & Co. in 2005, determined the 'return on investment' from doctor-led discussion groups was almost double the return on meetings led by the company's own sales force. According to the document, doctors who attended a lecture by another doctor wrote an additional $623.55 worth of prescriptions for the painkiller Vioxx over a 12-month period compared to doctors who did not attend a lecture. That can be compared to an increase of only $165.87 in Vioxx prescriptions by doctors who did not attend a lecture and met only with a salesperson."[1,3]

On the national level, legislation addressing these concerns has been enacted. The Physician Payments Sunshine Act created the Open Payments Program, which is administered by the Centers for Medicare and Medicaid Services (CMS). The program is designed to create greater transparency around the financial relationships between the pharmaceutical industry, physicians, and teaching hospitals. The Sunshine Act began on August 1, 2013 and requires certain pharmaceutical and device manufacturers to report payments or other transfers of value given to U.S. physicians and teaching hospitals. Reports are produced yearly, and the information is accessible to the public on the web. Manufacturers must report payments or value for the following: funding for research, travel, honoraria, speaking fees, and meals.

As a result of these actions, marketing dollars have shifted away from drug reps and physicians and now are spent directly on advertising to the consumers. The aim of this direct-to-consumer (DTC) advertising is for patients to learn of medications and ask for them by name at their physician's office. There has been a significant increase in drug advertisements on television. The United States is one of the few countries that still permits pharmaceutical advertising on television.

As a consumer it is important to keep in mind the influence the pharmaceutical companies can have over yourself and physicians in terms of advertising. When asking a physician about a medication, a good approach is to mention the medication and ask the physician of his or her experiences with the medication. Additionally, if your doctor is insistent on prescribing a certain medication, a good question to ask is there a less expensive alternative. In the world of medications, newer is not always necessarily better. Aspirin has been around for centuries and is a very effective treatment to lower both the risk of a heart attack as well as a stroke. Newer and more expensive medications are available but may not improve outcomes or do so minimally and at a substantially higher cost.

Given the costs of medications, they should be prescribed only if they work and continue to work. Medications should not be taken if they are supposed to work and no improvement is noted. For example, if an individual begins a new medication to lower blood pressure and no effect is noted, the medication should be discontinued and another class of medication should be tried.

Prescription

A prescription is a written order or message from a doctor to a pharmacist, therapist, or medical supplier. The prescription will direct him or her to dispense or initiate the use a medicine, therapy or medical equipment. Historically, prescriptions have been written on prescription paper. More recently, the federal government has encouraged prescribers to send the prescriptions electronically. Prescriptions may also be phoned into the pharmacy by a physician or their office staff.

Classifications

Medications can be classified or categorized based on a number of factors including mechanism of action, purpose, addiction potential, and risks to the fetus during pregnancy.

Drug Schedules

The Controlled Substances Act (CSA) created five schedules (classifications) based on the addictive potential of the medication. Two federal agencies, the Drug Enforcement Administration (DEA) and the Food and Drug Administration (FDA), determine which substances are added or removed from the various schedules.

Schedule I drugs, substances, or chemicals are defined as drugs with no currently accepted medical use and a high potential for abuse. They are felt to be the most dangerous drugs of all the drug schedules with potentially severe psychological or physical dependence. Some examples of schedule I drugs are heroin, LSD, marijuana, and ecstasy.

Schedule II drugs are defined as drugs with a high potential for abuse. Use may lead to severe psychological or physical dependence. These drugs are also considered potentially dangerous but have been shown to have medical value. Some examples of schedule II drugs are Adderall, cocaine, Demerol, Dilaudid, Lortab, methadone, OxyContin, Percocet, Ritalin, and Vicodin. It is unlawful to possess or take a controlled II substance without a prescription; it is also against the law to sell, share, or divert schedule II medications. Patients who are under a physician's care for substance II medications are required to be seen by the physician every 90 days. The prescriptions have historically been limited to a 30-day supply with no refills, although this regulation may be changing.

Schedule III-V drugs exhibit a lower potential for physical and psychological dependence and are outlined in table 6.1.

TABLE 6.1 SUMMARY OF CONTROLLED SUBSTANCE CATEGORIES

Category	Addiction Potential	Examples	Rx
I	Extremely high	Heroin, LSD, marijuana, and ecstasy	None
II	Very high	Hydrocodone, cocaine, Adderall, methadone, Dilaudid, Demerol, OxyContin, fentanyl, and Ritalin	30-day supply
III	Significant	T3 (Tylenol with codeine), ketamine, anabolic steroids, and testosterone	30-plus-day refills
IV	Reduced	Xanax, Soma, Valium, Ativan, Talwin, Ambien, and Tramadol	30-plus-day refills
V	Low	Robitussin AC, Lomotil, Lyrica, and Parepectolin	30-plus-day refills

Addiction

Abuse as defined by the CMS is the intentional nontherapeutic use of a drug, even once, to achieve a desired psychological or physiological effect. The CMS defines drug *addiction* as a cluster of behavioral, cognitive, and physiological phenomena that may include a strong desire to take the drug, difficulties in controlling drug use (e.g., continuing drug use despite harmful consequences, giving a higher priority to drug use than any other activities and obligations), and possible tolerance or physical dependence.

Addiction is felt to be a growing problem in America currently, which has caused federal and state programs to address this problem. Why is there such a problem? Medications used for pain (narcotics) have no ceiling effect, which means they can continue to be raised as the patient develops a greater tolerance. Tolerance is developed as the liver adapts to metabolizing the medication. In addition, there can be receptor changes at the level of the central nervous system (CNS) where the drugs interact and induce pleasurable feelings in certain centers of the brain with its use.

An additional factor regarding addiction is the prescribing of the narcotic medications for chronic nonmalignant (noncancerous) pain. The medications will help initially and then as the patient develops tolerance the medication dosage will need to be increased. After it is increased the pain will be improved for a time period and the medication will need increased once again, and the cycle will continue until a point where the prescribing physician may not feel comfortable increasing the dosage further. Narcotics are not medications that can be abruptly stopped since they will often lead to withdrawal. Withdrawal is not life threatening but can be an awful experience that some patients have described as the worst experience of their lives. This is a significant component as why getting patients off the medication can be so difficult. In order to get off the addictive medication the patient must want to get off the medication and will need to go through a slow taper of the medication dosage with education regarding withdrawal a necessary part of the plan.

Medications during Pregnancy

In addition to their potential addiction, medications are also classified according to their risks to the fetus if taken during pregnancy. Any female who is attempting to become or who is pregnant should inform her physician of her status and review any current medications she is taking or may plan to take.

Copay Structure

Most insurance products offer a tier system regarding payment for medications. The system will have the patient contribute to the cost of the medication by paying a certain amount of the medication, known as a copayment (copay). A three-tier system is the most common. Tier 1 medications include generic medications and have the lowest copayment or may not require a copay. Tier 2 medications are preferred brand-name medications associated with a higher copayment amount. Tier 3 medications are the nonpreferred medications and require the highest copay amount. The copay amounts have increased over the past few years. Different insurance carriers offer different preferred formularies (medications that are covered at a tier 1 or 2 level in the plan). If you have a choice in selecting your insurance plan, knowing their formulary and matching it to your medication needs may be financially beneficial.

Savings

Most people who are shopping for a car do not buy the first automobile they see, but they shop around and compare the prices to get the best deals. Most patients, however, do not shop around for medications. There is a misconception that their insurance plan will cover the entire cost of the medication. This may be true for tier 1 medications, but the medication portion of the insurance plan may require the patient to pay for a percentage of the cost of the medication. For example, if a 30-day supply of your cholesterol medication costs $150 at pharmacy A and $50 dollars at pharmacy B, and you are required to pay 30% of the costs, under your insurance plan, you could save $30 by filling the prescription at pharmacy B. A convenient way to price check can be done by downloading a smart phone application that compares medication prices. There are applications for smart phones that have you enter the medication and your zip code, and they will compare the local pharmacies and show you the pricing at each one. Two more popular apps that do this are LowestMED and Good Rx. Saving money on medication can be significant. I have personally informed patients and students of this and they have saved between $15–$300 per month!

Generic Medications

Generic medications are a way to substantially reduce the costs associated with prescriptions. Generic medications are *bioequivalent* (identical) to brand name drugs. They are produced after the patent on the new medication has expired. According to the FDA the patent is currently at 20 years from the date on which the application for the patent was filed in the United States. The generics are produced in the same dosage amount and quality as the brand medication. They are sold at discounted prices since there is likely no need for marketing and advertising costs associated with the drug.

Over-the-Counter Medications

Over-the-counter medications (OTC) are sold directly to the consumer. No prescription is necessary to obtain these medications. The anti-inflammatory medicines for arthritis pain are the most commonly used OTC medication. It is important to remember that OTC medications can have significant side effects and can certainly interact with prescription medications one may be taking. It is important to let your physician know what medications you are taking, including OTC medications. No medication is completely free of side effects.

CLINICAL PEARL

It may be surprising to see marijuana as a schedule I drug. Schedule I drugs are illegal at the federal level but are legal to use in certain states for medical and even recreation use. The Drug Enforcement Administration (DEA) recently, in August 2016, reaffirmed its stance on marijuana being a schedule I drug. Certain states were hoping for a drop to a schedule II drug; however, the

DEA did permit expanded research into the medical effects of marijuana. The federal law supersedes state laws. The DEA has not taken action against the states that have legalized marijuana for medical or recreational use. The Justice Department has reserved its right to challenge state laws if public health problems occur in the states that have legalized marijuana.

Resources

Centers for Medicare and Medicaid Services: Open payments is a national disclosure program that promotes a transparent and accountable health care system by making the financial relationships between applicable manufacturers (pharmaceuticals), medical organizations, and health care providers available to the public: https://www.cms.gov/openpayments/

Gwen Olsen: Site founded by Gwen Olsen former pharmaceutical rep, devoted to educating the public in regards to medications and fostered improved outcomes: http://gwenolsen.com/

Food and Drug Administration: Website that reviews the process of medication approval from the FDA and serves to expand the consumers knowledge of getting the medication to the public: https://www.fda.gov/forpatients/approvals/drugs/ucm405622.htm

World Health Organization: Home site of the organization devoted to improving global health: http://www.who.int/en/

U.S. Food and Drug Administration: Link is to a manual detailing basic concepts regarding controlled substances and addiction; the definition section of the manual does a great job of comparing and defining the various terms associated with addiction: https://www.fda.gov/downloads/AboutFDA/ReportsManualsForms/StaffPoliciesandProcedures/ucm073580.pdf

Endnotes

1. WHO Medicines Strategy: Framework or Action in Essential Drugs and Medicines Policy 2000–2003. Geneva: WHO, 200 (WHO/EDM/2000.1).

2. Global Comparative Pharmaceutical Expenditures with related reference information. *Health Economics and Drugs, EDM Series* no. 3 Geneva: WHO, 2000 (WHO/EDM/2000.3).

3. Scott Hensley and Barbara Martinez, "To Sell Their Drugs, Companies Increasingly Rely on Doctors: For $750 and Up, Physicians Tell Peers About Products; Talks Called Educational," *Wall Street Journal,* July 2005 Wall Street Journal 2005 July 15; p. A1, A2.

Chapter 7

Nutrition and Health

Trying to write a chapter on nutrition and health information for consumers and limit it to less than a dozen pages is a formidable if not an impossible task. Classes on nutrition principles can easily last an entire semester, with textbooks exceeding hundreds of pages. This chapter serves to highlight basic concepts of nutrition and provide an overview of the common pitfalls that can adversely affect one's health.

Nutrition

Nutrition, as defined by Oxford Dictionaries, is the process of providing or obtaining the food necessary for health and growth. The food we ingest provides us with energy to grow and maintain our bodies. Food intake is denoted in terms of calories. The calorie is a measurement of energy. We like to classify calories as both consumed and expended (burned). One's diet is composed of the calories consumed, and the calories burned relates to that individual's activity.

If our input is greater than our output we *gain* weight, and if our output is greater than our input we *lose* weight. When our intake or input exceeds our output, our body converts the calories into fat.

One pound of fat is equivalent to 3,500 calories. So, if an individual's intake is greater than his or her output by 3,500 calories for the week, one pound of fat is added to the body. Fat is used by our body to store excess energy, which can be burned at a later time if needed. However, if that excess fat is not burned, additional fat continues to get added.

In order to lose one pound of weight (fat) in one week, your weekly intake needs to be less than your output by 3,500 calories. That breaks down to a difference of 500 calories a day. You either need to take in 500 calories less a day or need to expend 500 calories more in a day or some combination of the two. There are three ways the body will expend energy: basal metabolic rate, thermic effect of food, and physical activity or exercise.

Basal Metabolic Rate

The basal metabolic rate (BMR) is the amount of energy needed to maintain a resting state and carry out basic metabolic functions of the body. This energy expenditure occurs when the body is at rest. Energy is required to maintain your body at 98.6°F, despite fluctuations in the ambient temperature. The body needs energy to enable the lungs to breathe and the heart to beat continuously. The BMR accounts for approximately 60% of the daily energy expenditures for the day.

Some of the issues with weight gain are related to age. We know that as we age our weight can easily climb. One aspect of this weight gain is related to the BMR. BMR decreases with age. One study found total energy expenditure fell by approximately 150,000 calories per decade. The study concluded this progressive decline in BMR and total energy expenditure has implications for defining dietary energy requirements at different stages of adult life.[1] In short, you cannot eat like you did when you were younger without likely gaining weight.

Thermic Effect of Food (TEF)

The thermic effect of food (TEF) is another way the body expends energy. The TEF is defined as the increase in metabolic rate after ingestion of a meal.[2] This is energy used to digest, absorb, and metabolize food. The energy is higher for digestion of complex carbohydrates and protein than it is for fat. The TEF accounts for about 8% of the total energy expenditures. The TEF varies with different temperatures of food/water intake. More energy is expended when one drinks a cup of ice water compared to an equivalent amount of room temperature water, but the energy expenditure is not truly significant. To put it simply, no you will not lose weight by drinking ice water all the time.

Exercise

The remaining way our bodies burn calories is through exercise, and this topic will be extensively reviewed in the next chapter of the book. The exercise aspect has been reported to account for the remaining 32% of the total energy expenditure. The amount of energy used or burned depends of the specific activity or exercise. As BMR decreases with age, so do activity levels and the ability to burn calories ingested, once again leading to difficulties with weight gain.

Input

The other half of the weight gain/loss balance is intake or input. This refers to the food and liquids that are consumed. Each of the basic nutrients contain different calorie amounts. Carbohydrates and proteins each contain 4 calories each per gram, fats contain 9 calories per gram, and alcohol 7 calories per gram. Alcohol is sometimes referred to as "empty calories" as it contains no nutritional value.

Carbohydrates

Carbohydrates are nutrients that provide the body with energy, and they can be further divided into simple carbohydrates and complex carbohydrates. *Complex carbohydrates* are also known as starches. *Simple carbohydrates* are sugars. Naturally occurring sugars include glucose and fructose. Simple carbohydrates are found naturally in fruits and milk but can also be processed into candy, syrups, and soft/fruit drinks. Refined sugars may be thought of as "empty calories" since they are not associated with vitamins and minerals. Simple carbohydrates and their high glycemic index will raise blood sugar levels quicker and higher than any other type of food.

Complex carbohydrates are also composed of sugar molecules, although the molecules are joined in long chains. In contrast to simple carbohydrates, complex carbohydrates provide important minerals and vitamins for the body. Complex carbohydrates, being composed of sugars, will be broken down by the body to be used as energy or converted to glycogen for storage in the liver. This conversion takes longer and is associated with a lower glycemic index than simple carbohydrates.

Fiber may be found within certain complex carbohydrates. Fiber may be further broken down into soluble and insoluble types. Soluble fiber works to improve blood sugar levels and helps to lower cholesterol levels. It is found in beans, lentils, nuts, and oat bran. As soluble fiber passes through the digestive system it attracts water, helping to slow digestion and soften the stool. This aids in treating constipation-related issues. Insoluble fiber is found in whole grains, vegetables, and wheat bran.

Protein

Protein is obtained from both animal and plant sources. It is used for energy and helps build and support the cells of the body.

Proteins are made up of thousands of amino acids that are chained together. The amino acids are building blocks for our muscles, skin, bones, and internal organs. Proteins are also used by our body to support our immune system. They are needed for the production of enzymes and hormones by the body. Proteins are a necessary part of our diet. Foods that are good sources of protein include meat, fish, chicken, eggs, milk, beans, and soy.

Fats

Fats are an essential part of our diet. Our bodies require fats to construct cell membranes, insulate nerves, produce hormones, and absorb vitamins. Fats are more difficult to digest than carbohydrates. There are two main types of fats: *saturated* fats and *unsaturated* fats. The unsaturated fats can further be subdivided into *monounsaturated* fats and *polyunsaturated* fats.

Saturated Fats

Saturated fats are found primarily from animal sources but not exclusively. Sources may include cheese, whole milk, bacon, beef, and pork. Historically, these fats have been considered "bad fats" and were felt to contribute to cardiovascular disease and specifically strokes and heart attacks. Although, a meta-analysis done in 2010 followed 347,000 subjects over a 5–23-year time period found no such evidence that dietary saturated fat was associated with an increased risk of coronary heart disease or cardiovascular disease.[3]

Additional studies have looked to see if any health benefits occur with a reduction of saturated fats in the diet. They were able to conclude that by replacing 5% of saturated fats in one's diet with polyunsaturated fat, the risk of coronary artery disease was lowered by about 10%.[4] It is for this reason the American Heart Association recommends that the intake of saturated fats be limited to no more than 7% of total intake.[5]

Monounsaturated Fats

Monounsaturated fats are found from plant sources. Avocados, almonds, and pumpkin seeds are all foods that contain a significant amount of monounsaturated fat. These fats along with polyunsaturated fats are considered "good fats." Research has shown that partial substitution of carbohydrate with either protein or monounsaturated fat can further lower blood pressure, improve lipid levels, and reduce estimated cardiovascular risk.[6] The American Heart Association suggests that 8–10 percent of daily calories should come from polyunsaturated fats.

Polyunsaturated Fats

Polyunsaturated fats are also considered "good fats." Salmon, walnuts, and sunflower oil are all good sources of polyunsaturated fats. Polyunsaturated fats are also sources of omega 3 and omega 6 fatty acids. These are both essential fatty acids that the body needs but cannot produce on its own. Omega 3 fatty acids are found specifically from fish and omega 6 fatty acids from plant sources. Research has suggested benefits of increasing the intake of both essential fatty acids, particularly omega 3, that are secondary from their anti-inflammatory effects.[7]

Caloric Density

Calorie counting can be done to know the exact daily intake of calories. Another factor to keep in mind is the caloric density of food we ingest. Certain foods are very dense with calories. These foods will contain a large amount of calories in a small weight of food. Foods that are low in calorie density will tend to be larger in size. This can help with satiety (feeling full) and gastric distension, giving one a feeling of being full after eating. For example, cheese is a food that has a high caloric density, while an apple has a low caloric density. One can eat a bite-size piece of cheese or opt for two apples. Their calories are equal, but the satiety with eating one-bite size piece of cheese is much different than 2 apples. Some of the recommended daily dietary recommendations account for calorie density.

Concern

The rate of obesity in the United States continues to present a major medical problem for the country on a national scale. On an individual level, obesity and excessive weight is associated with a number of medical problems. Increased rates of heart disease, diabetes, high blood pressure, cancer, and arthritis are associated with obesity. A number of factors have played a role in the obesity problem. The solution to this problem needs to address multiple issues and areas of concern. Educating the public should create a better awareness and allow for healthier choices to be made.

Education

It is important to understand the basics of calories and the amount of calories that are associated with the foods we eat. Foods that are bought in a store all contain caloric and nutritional information. But, according to the FDA, Americans eat and drink about 33% of their calories away from home. In 2018, a statute was passed requiring nutrition labeling in chain restaurants. The information posted must include calorie information as it relates to suggested daily caloric intake. More detailed information including the break-down of fats, carbohydrates, fiber, sugar, and protein will be made available in writing upon request.

Awareness

The caloric information should certainly help with education. Knowing the information is helpful, but having a strong awareness of the information should help further. One may hear the com-mon phrase "I know it's bad for me but …" What exactly does bad mean? Are we aware as consumers of what exactly bad is and what are the consequences of making such choices?

The development of late onset or type 2 diabetes is well known to be linked to obesity. Research has also found additional risk factors: soft drinks and *fruit drinks*. You may have thought your apple or orange juice to be healthy, but one study examined 50,000 female subjects over a nine-year period and found women consuming one or more sugar-sweetened soft drinks per day had a relative risk of type 2 diabetes that is 1.83 times greater than those who consumed less than one of these beverages per month.[8] Similarly, consumption of fruit punch was associated with increased diabetes risk that is two times greater than those who did not consume fruit punch.[9] This study was published in 2004. Another study in African American females to evaluate the risks of both soft drinks and fruit juice found consumption of two or more soft drinks increased the risk to develop diabetes by 28%, and fruit juice consumption increased the risk by 30%.[10] This study was published in 2008. These studies were published more than a decade ago, yet this is likely the first time you are learning this information.

Oversize

Most people when purchasing an item want to get their money's worth. When this concept is applied to food the end result may not always be in your best interest. For example, at certain fast food chains and gas/convenience stores they charge the same the price for a small, medium, large, or extra-large soft drink. The price may be the same, but the calories and amount of sugar contained in the different sizes is not.

Portions have also increased over the years in the United States. What we think of a portion now has changed dramatically. According to the NIH, "Average portion sizes have grown so much over the past 20 years that sometimes the plate arrives and there's enough food for two or even three people on it. Growing portion sizes are changing what Americans think of as a 'normal' portion at home too. This is known as 'portion distortion.'"[11] Some examples include a bagel twenty years ago being 3 inches in diameter and containing 140 calories. Today's bagel averages 6 inches in diameter and contains 350 calories. The average soda was once 6.5 ounces and contained 82 calories, yet today's soda averages 20 ounces and 250 calories. Table 7.1 outlines the differences.

TABLE 7.1 COMPARISON OF PORTIONS AND CALORIES TWENTY YEARS AGO TO PRESENT DAY

	20 Years Ago		*Today*	
	Portion	Calories	Portion	Calories
Bagel	3" diameter	140	6" diameter	350
Cheeseburger	1	333	1	590
Spaghetti w/meatballs	1 cup sauce 3 small meatballs	500	2 cups sauce 3 large meatballs	1,020
Soda	6.5 ounces	82	20 ounces	250
Blueberry muffin	1.5 ounces	210	5 ounces	500

Recommendations

The government has made recommendations regarding daily calorie intake and the amounts of carbohydrates, protein, and fats in the diet. These recommendations are based on research studies that have evaluated the effects of certain foods on our health and wellbeing. There are also recommendations for the amounts of the particular food groups: breads, meats, oils, fruits, and vegetables. The daily USDA recommendations are 6–11 servings of bread, cereal, rice, and pasta, 3–5 servings of the vegetable group, 2–4 servings of the fruit group, 2–3 servings of the milk, cheese and yogurt group, and 2–3 servings of meat, poultry, fish, dry beans, eggs and nuts, with sparing use of fats, oils, and sweets.

CLINICAL PEARL

Much has been made out of the health concerns of high fructose corn syrup. Companies have made a point to advertise their products with various slogans: "Contains NO high fructose corn syrup" or "Made with Natural Sugar." There is no significant difference between high fructose corn syrup and table sugar (sucrose). Sucrose is made up of 50% glucose and 50% fructose. High-fructose corn syrup is also made up of a glucose/fructose mixture either in a 58:42 or a 45:55 ratio. What matters more is the total amount of the sugar in the food product.

Resources

Nutrition.gov: USDA-sponsored website that offers credible information for consumers to make informed and healthful eating choices: www.nutrition.gov

American Diabetes Association: Home page of the association dedicated to informing and improving individuals and family members with diabetes: http://www.diabetes.org/

U.S. Food and Drug Administration: Site of the FDA to inform consumers the background of labeling and packaging of foods: www.fda.gov/food/ingredientspackaginglabeling

Endnotes

1. Susan B. Roberts and Gerard E. Dallal, "Energy Requirements and Aging," *Public Health Nutrition* 8, no. 7A (2005): 1028–1036.
2. G. W. Reed and James O. Hill, "Measuring the Thermic Effect of Food," *American Journal of Clinical Nutrition* 63, no. 2 (1996): 164–169.
3. Patty W. Siri-Tarino, Qi Sun, Frank B. Hu, and Ronald M. Krauss, "Meta-Analysis of Prospective Cohort Studies Evaluating the

Association of Saturated Fat with Cardiovascular Disease," *American Journal of Clinical Nutrition* 91, no. 3 (2010): 535–546.

4. Renata Micha and Darioush Mozaffarian, "Saturated Fat and Cardiometabolic Risk Factors, Coronary Heart Disease, Stroke, and Diabetes: A Fresh Look at the Evidence," *Lipids* 45, no. 10 (2010): 893–905.

5. Alice H. Lichtenstein et al., "Diet and Lifestyle Recommendations Revision 2006: A Scientific Statement from the American Heart Association Nutrition Committee," *Circulation* 114, no. 1 (2006): 82–96.

6. Lawrence J. Appel et al., "Effects of Protein, Monounsaturated Fat, and Carbohydrate Intake on Blood Pressure and Serum Lipids: Results of the OmniHeart Randomized Trial," *Journal of the American Medical Association* 294, no. 19 (2005): 2455–2464.

7. William Harris, "Omega-6 and Omega-3 Fatty Acids: Partners in Prevention," *Current Opinion in Clinical Nutrition and Metabolic Care* 13, no. 2 (2010): 125–129, doi:10.1097/MCO.0b013e3283357242.

8. Matthias B. Schulze et al., "Sugar-Sweetened Beverages, Weight Gain, and Incidence of Type 2 Diabetes in Young and Middle-Aged Women," *Journal of the American Medical Association* 292, no. 8 (2004): 927–934.

9. Julie R. Palmer et al., "Sugar-Sweetened Beverages and Incidence of Type 2 Diabetes Mellitus in African American Women," *Archives of Internal Medicine* 168, no. 14 (2008): 1487–1492, doi:10.1001/archinte.168.14.1487.

10. Josefin Edwall Löfvenborg et al., "Sweetened Beverage Intake and Risk of Latent Autoimmune Diabetes in Adults and Type 2 Diabetes," *European Journal of Endocrinology* 175, no. 6 (2016): 605–614.

11. "Portion Distortion." *National Heart, Lung, and Blood Institute*, last modified April 1, 2015. https://www.nhlbi.nih.gov/health/educational/wecan/eat-right/portion-distortion.htm

Chapter 8

Exercise and Related Topics

For centuries mankind has searched for the "fountain of youth." It was searched extensively by Ponce de León in the area that is now Florida. The mythical fountain has never been found, although one may argue the benefits of exercise can in some way be considered a fountain of youth. This chapter will outline the various types of exercise to both educate and inspire.

Exercise

Exercise can be described as physical activity for the purpose of improving or sustaining one's health. There are four main types of exercise: endurance, strength, balance, and flexibility. Each type has different benefits to improving one's health or fitness. A combination of the different types will provide you with the most health benefits. If the focus is entirely on strength, deficits in flexibility may prove problematic. Similarly, balance improvements will likely require strength improvements.

Endurance

Endurance exercises are activities that focus on improving one's aerobic (oxygen-related) capacity. Aerobic exercises focus on improving the oxygen-carrying capacity of the body. We obtain oxygen when we breathe; the oxygen enters the red blood cells (RBC) during an exchange of oxygen for carbon dioxide in the lungs. The heart then pumps the oxygenated blood throughout our body for use in all cells. Endurance exercise works to improve efficiency of the lungs and heart.

Beginning an endurance program is generally the hardest step. Some may have difficulty carving out time secondary to a busy schedule, in others the hardest part is to *initiate* a program. In most individuals, medical clearance is not required to initiate a program. However, there are certain patient demographics that should obtain physician clearance before beginning an exercise program. It is recommended by the American College of Sports Medicine to see your physician prior to starting an exercise program if two or more of the following conditions apply to your situation: age greater than 35, high blood pressure, high cholesterol, diabetes, current or recent (within past six months) smoking, or a family history of heart disease in family members before the age of 60. If you are unsure it is always best to check with your physician.

Heart rate (HR) is defined as the number of heart beats (contractions) in one minute of time. It is usually expressed as beats per minute (bpm). One can take their HR by feeling for changes in the pressure of their arteries (pulse). This is most commonly done by measuring the pulse at the wrist. The number of pulsations are then counted over a one-minute time period. You can also estimate your pulse by timing over a thirty-second time period and doubling the number. Recently, smart phones and exercise watches have incorporated technologies to measure one's pulse, too.

The maximum HR is the maximum number of heart beats per minute during exercise. The formula to determine maximum HR is 220-age of the individual. For example, the maximum HR in a 60-year-old is 220-60 = 160 bpm. It is recommended not to exceed this value during exercise. Most aerobic or endurance exercise is performed at a level of 80% of the maximum heart rate. Let's figure out the target heart rate for a 40-year-old who wishes to exercise at the 80% level. This is calculated by knowing the maximum HR is 220-40 (their age) = 180 and then multiplying the 180 × 0.80 (80% level) = 144 bpm. This is the target HR to maintain during the exercise routine that will result in improving one's fitness.

Endurance exercises include running, cycling, and swimming, any of which can improve fitness in individuals. When the body is engaged in this type of exercise for a sustained period of time it releases *endorphins*. Endorphins are natural chemicals produced by the body that are similar to morphine. They can help to ease pain and improve mood in those who exercise regularly, producing the "runner's high."

Strength

Strength training refers to exercises that improve muscle power and efficiency. Muscles work by contracting or shortening their length. They typically cross a joint of the body and occasionally two joints. The end of the muscle is known as a tendon and the tendon connects the muscle to a bone. Contraction or shortening of the muscle will produce movement of the bone and joint. Muscles can act on a limb as a flexor or as an extensor. Flexors flex the extremity, while extensors act in an opposite direction to extend them. The biceps will contract, and this will result in flexion of the elbow. Then the opposing (antagonist) muscle group, the triceps, will contract and extend the elbow.

There are different types of contractions muscles can engage in. These contractions are known as isotonic, isometric, and isokinetic. The prefix "iso" translates into equal.

Isotonic contractions maintain constant tension in the muscle as the muscle changes length. This can occur only when a muscle's maximal force of contraction exceeds the total load on the muscle.[1] Isotonic muscle contractions can be concentric or eccentric. Concentric contractions occur when the muscle shortens. In contrast, eccentric contractions occur when the muscle lengthens. An example of a concentric contraction is using a dumbbell to do a biceps curl; as the weight is lifted up, the biceps concentrically contract, flexing the elbow and lifting the weight. As the weight is lowered, the biceps will contract eccentrically, slowly lowering the weight. If the biceps did not eccentrically contract, the weight would suddenly drop. Eccentric exercises are associated with greater strength gains.

Isometric contractions generate force without changing the length of the muscle. This is typical of muscles found in the hands and forearm: muscles do not change length, and joints are not moved, so force for grip is sufficient.[2] An example of this occurs when performing a chin up, when one holds his or her position at the top before he or she begins to lower. The muscles in this position are performing an isometric contraction; there is no movement, but they are active in maintaining a static position.

The third and final type of muscle contraction is an *isokinetic* contraction. This type of contraction is performed when the limb is in constant motion and variable resistance is applied. This type of exercise will engage in contracting your muscles with movement of your limb. An example of this muscle is when one uses a stationary cycle. His or her movement is maintained it in a constant motion with the potential for variable resistance.

Muscles function to move our extremities. They are also responsible for controlling our core to help maintain our balance.

Balance

One may not necessarily think of improving balance as an exercise, but maintaining balance is crucial especially as we age. Impaired balance in the elderly may result in a hip fracture, which can have devastating consequences. Balance is like any other skill one may learn; you can either use it or lose it. Specific exercises to safely challenge balance can improve both balance and coordination. These improvements can reduce risk of falls while serving to improve one's core strength.

Tai chi is an ancient Chinese discipline that focuses on the mind and body. The gentle movements will emphasize certain postures and place additional mental focus on breathing and relaxation. The movements or sets of movements are typically practiced while standing. Studies have examined the potential positive effects of tai chi.

One study found that older people who took part in a 15-week tai chi program reduced their risk of multiple falls by 47.5 percent.[3]

Another study showed tai chi to improve balance and strength among older people. These improvements, particularly in strength, were preserved over a six-month period in participants who did the tai chi exercises.[4]

Flexibility

Another type of exercise are those directed at improving flexibility. Flexibility exercises stretch muscles and their associated tendons. These exercises allow for improved movements as well as promoting a maximal range of motion of joints in the body. Improving one's flexibility may be an initial first step in addressing back pain. Low back pain is commonly seen in conjunction with hamstring tightness. The hamstrings are found in the posterior thigh region of the body, and they connect the pelvic area to an area just below the knees. The hamstrings function to flex our knees. Back posture is improved with stretching of the hamstrings, and back pain is increased with tightness in the hamstrings. Other muscles that develop tightness and inflexibilities are the neck muscles, shoulder muscles, and hip muscles. The tightness can contribute to a cycle of increased pain and thus decreased flexibilities may lead to increased pain and so forth.

Flexibility exercises will have the most benefit if done when the muscles are warm and not cold. Stretching a muscle will have the greatest benefit if done after the 3-mile run and not before the run. After the run the muscles are considered warmed up. Additionally, a moist heating pad can be applied to a muscle for 20 minutes prior to the stretch. After one completes a workout, or following a warm shower/bath are other good opportunities to stretch muscles.

Recommendations

The U.S. government recommends adults get at least 2.5 hours of moderate-intensity aerobic exercise each week or one hour and

15 minutes of vigorous-intensity activity, or a combination of both. It is also recommended that adults also engage in muscle-strengthening activities twice per week. These recommendations are based on the findings of multiple research studies. Given the hectic pace of our lives today, it is important that one makes time for exercise. Simply knowing the recommendations does not lend itself to any health benefits.

Benefits

The benefits of exercise are numerous. In general terms the benefits fall into four categories: enhancing function, maintaining reserve capacities, preventing disease, and ameliorating the effects of age and chronic disease.[5] Specifically exercise has shown to do the following: reduce the risk of heart attack, reduce the risk of a stroke, reduce the risk of breast cancer, reduce the risk of colon cancer, reduce the risk of prostate cancer, reduce the risk of endometrium cancer, reduce anxiety, reduce depression, reduce risk of dementia, reduce the risk of falls, reduce risk of osteoporosis, elevate mood, increase intellectual functioning, improve self-esteem, improve weight control, improve Parkinson's disease, improve pain of fibromyalgia, and improve bone mass.[6-11]

There was probably no better champion for exercise than Jack LaLanne. He was a true believer in the value and importance of exercise and fitness. He promoted healthy living on television and by his lifestyle. He completed extraordinary feats which included the following: At age 45, he completed 1,000 pushups and 1,000 chin-ups in 1 hour and 22 minutes; at age 60 he swam from Alcatraz Island to Fisherman's Wharf handcuffed, shackled, and towing a 1,000-pound boat; and at the age of 70, handcuffed, shackled, and fighting strong winds and currents, he towed seventy boats with seventy people from the Queen's Way Bridge in the Long Beach Harbor to the Queen Mary, a distance of 1.5 miles. Not everyone can aspire to that level of fitness, but getting started and maintaining a regular exercise program may be the closest one can get to the fountain of youth.

CLINICAL PEARL

There is some confusion as when to use ice or heat for injuries. Ice should be applied for immediate (acute) injuries, as it reduces blood flow and the inflammatory cascade. It is recommend to apply ice for at least 20 minutes to help with acute swelling and pain for the first 72 hours after an injury. Ice is also very helpful in treating a muscle cramp. Ice will cool the muscle, and this will allow the muscle to relax and arrest the cramp. Heat is used to treat muscle soreness and can be applied to the area for 20 minutes. Heat can also be used after the initial 72 hours after an acute injury to promote blood flow and allow for healing of the injury.

Resources

Centers for Disease Control and Prevention: CDC-sponsored site on the recommendations and different types of exercises with links to the proven health benefits: https://www.cdc.gov/physicalactivity/basics/adults/index.htm

Jack LaLanne: Website devoted to the "godfather of modern fitness"; this site reviews his basic principles and details the incredible feats he achieved throughout his life. It is a very inspiring site to promote the benefits of fitness: http://jacklalanne.com

Endnotes

1. "Control of Muscle Tension," *Lumen*, accessed June 3, 2019, https://courses.lumenlearning.com/boundless-ap/chapter/control-of-muscle-tension/.
2. Ibid.
3. Steven L. Wolf et al., "Reducing Frailty and Falls in Older Persons: An investigation of Tai Chi and Computerized Balance Training," *Journal of the American Geriatric Society* 44, no. 5 (1996): 489–97.

4. Leslie Wolfson et al., "Balance and Strength Training in Older Adults: Intervention Gains and Tai Chi Maintenance," *Journal of the American Geriatric Society* 44, no. 5 (1996): 498–506.

5. Peter H. Fentem, "ABC of Sports Medicine: Benefits of Exercise in Health and Disease," BMJ 308 (1994): 1291.

6. Kate E. Cruise et al., "Exercise and Parkinson's: Benefits for Cognition and Quality of Life". Acta Neurologica Scandinavica, 123 (2011): 13–19, doi:10.1111/j.1600-0404.2010.01338.x.

7. Julie Anthony, "Psychologic Aspects of Exercise," Clinics in Sports Medicine 10, no. 1 (1991): 171–180.

8. Harri Vainio and Franca Bianchini, *Weight Control and Physical Activity*, Vol. 6 (Lyon, France: International Agency for Research Cancer Press, 2002).

9. Alpa V. Patel et al., "Obesity, Recreational Physical Activity, and Risk of Pancreatic Cancer in a Large U.S. Cohort," *Cancer Epidemiology, Biomarkers and Prevention* 14, no. 2 (2005): 459–466.

10. Alpa V. Patel et al., "Recreational Physical Activity and Risk of Postmenopausal Breast Cancer in a Large Cohort of U.S. Women," *Cancer Causes & Control* 14, no. 6 (2003): 519–529.

11. Arthur C. Santora, II, "Role of Nutrition and Exercise in Osteoporosis," *American Journal of Medicine* 82, no. 1 (1987): 73–9.

Chapter 9

Mental Health and Related Therapies

Health is dependent on both physical and mental aspects. Mental health is a very an important area of medicine that has been historically under addressed despite its prevalence. According to the National Institute of Mental Health nearly one in five adults live with a mental illness. The importance of recognizing a mental health condition and receiving appropriate treatment can be paramount in improving one's and loved ones' quality of life.

Psychiatrist

A psychiatrist is a physician who completed a psychiatry residency and specializes in the diagnosis and treatment of mental disorders. *Psychiatrists* will examine patients and determine whether the patient's symptoms are the result of a physical/mental aliment or combination of both. Diagnostic or specifically laboratory tests may need to be done to evaluate the possibility of a metabolic cause. An example of this is mercury poisoning. Elevated levels of mercury in the body can cause a myriad of symptoms which may include mood swings, irritability, insomnia (inability to sleep), and abnormal sensations, all of which can be seen with depression. The psychiatrist will establish a treatment plan, which may include prescribing a medication and/or having the patient see a psychologist or mental health counselor for services.

Mental Health Counselor

A mental health counselor is a health care professional who has attained a master's-level degree and is trained in counseling. Mental health counselors provide guidance and support to individuals and family in regards to mental health issues. They provide traditional psychotherapy with a problem-solving approach toward effective change. Clinical mental health counseling has national standards for education, training, and clinical practice.

Psychologist

A *psychologist* is typically a professional who has attained a doctorate degree and specializes in mental health issues. Psychologists are trained to diagnose and treat mental, emotional, and behavioral disorders. They are trained in various techniques and counseling to effectively treat patients. They may also engage in diagnostic cognitive testing to better understand issues to provide a novel approach to treat the problem. They provide services at either the individual, family, or group level. They may also provide patients with programs to work on behavior modification. Psychologists *do not* prescribe medications. The duties of a psychologist will depend on the specific type of training of the psychologist as well as the environment of practice.

Clinical psychologists are trained to diagnose and treat mental, emotional, and behavioral disorders. They may help individuals with short-term personal issues (e.g., the loss of a spouse or loved one). They may also see patients on a long-term basis for chronic behavioral or mental issues. These may include depression or an anxiety disorder. They are trained in various techniques and counseling to effectively treat clients. They may also engage in diagnostic cognitive testing to better understand the issues in order to address problems. Psychologists run group sessions to help with treatment. They may design and provide patients with programs to work on behavior modification.

Neuropsychologists are a specialized subset of clinical psychologists who study the effects of brain injuries/disease, developmental disorders, or mental health conditions on behavior and thinking. They test patients with various cognitive conditions to determine the deficits on thinking. Neuropsychologists may perform extensive testing to better understand the effects of a concussion, stroke, or attention deficit hyperactivity disorder (ADHD). Understanding the problematic areas can allow for an appropriate treatment plan.

Counseling psychologists help patients deal with and understand emotional and relationship problems. They may address problematic relationships that occur at home. Sometimes they may need to address problems that occur secondary to stressors in the workplace. They will counsel patients to help manage their concerns. The management plan may include providing patients with visual imagery techniques or biofeedback.

Developmental psychologists will specifically address the psychological developmental progress. They can treat patients throughout their lifetime. The developmental psychologist may be employed by a school. They may address student learning and behavioral problems, design and implement performance plans, evaluate performances, and counsel students/families. They also may consult with other school-based professionals to suggest improvements to teaching, learning, and administrative strategies. These psychologists will work with the student and the school to establish an appropriate treatment program. They may also work with elderly patients focusing on problems associated with aging. These problems include dementia or physical impairments that may affect individuals from an emotional standpoint.

Treatment Options

Mental health issues, including depression and anxiety, can commonly be treated by a patient's primary care provider. More complex mental health issues may involve treatment with a psychiatrist, psychologist, and mental health counselor. Insurance typically covers mental health provider care and treatment, similar to typical medical services.

Diagnostic and Statistical Manual of Mental Disorders

The *Diagnostic and Statistical Manual of Mental Disorders*, fifth edition (DSM-5) is the standard guide used by mental health experts for the diagnosis of various mental health problems. It is published by the American Psychiatric Association. They state the DSM-5 is the product of more than 10 years of work by hundreds of international experts in all aspects of mental health. The manual is updated regularly when research is produced that allows a better understanding of the various mental disorders. Some of the more common disorders will be reviewed next. The list is by no means comprehensive but rather some of the more common conditions that affect consumers, with a basic explanation to allow for a better understanding and give direction for treatment options.

Autism

Autism is a neurodevelopmental disorder for dysfunctions with the development of the central nervous system. The dysfunctions can manifest as a variety of problems and may include impairments in language or communication, impairments in motor function, and neuropsychiatric problems. Since the development of the central nervous system is involved, the noted difficulties may be apparent in infancy or childhood. Autism spectrum disorder (ASD) is an example of a neurodevelopmental disorder. The *spectrum* designation refers to the fact that a range of symptoms can be seen within this diagnosis. Individuals with ASD can exhibit difficulties with conversation, an intense focus on certain subjects/details/facts, sensitivity to sensory input (sound, clothing, temperature), and reporting certain words or phrases (echolalia). The cause of ASD is unknown, although genetics and environmental causes are felt to play a role. The CDC estimates the incidence of ASD is 1.69% in children. Early intervention and treatment have been shown to lead to better results. These may include medications, behavior, and communication therapies.

Schizophrenia

Schizophrenia, as described by the National Institute of Mental Health, is a chronic and severe mental disorder that affects how a person thinks, feels, and behaves. People with schizophrenia are often described as losing touch with reality. Schizophrenia is not a condition of having split or multiple personalities. This misconception likely originated from the movie *Psycho*. Schizophrenia is a chronic condition requiring lifelong treatment.

Individuals with schizophrenia often exhibit symptoms that are classified as either positive or negative. Positive symptoms are typically psychotic in nature and those that appear to reflect an excess or distortion of normal functions. The diagnosis of schizophrenia, according to DSM-5, requires at least a one-month duration of two or more positive symptoms. Positive symptoms may include hallucinations, delusions, and thought/movement disorders.

Hallucinations will describe when one sees or hears something that does not exist. Hallucinations can be in any of the senses but hearing voices (auditory hallucinations) are the most common type. Delusions refer to false beliefs that are not based in reality. Thought disorders may be observed as communication that is disjointed, commonly referred to as "world salad." Movement disorders are agitated body movements.

Negative symptoms typically will affect emotions and behaviors. Negative symptoms include the following: flat affect (depression), difficulty staying on task, and anhedonia (reduced feelings of pleasure). Negative symptoms often persist in the lives of people with schizophrenia during periods of low or absent positive symptoms.

Schizophrenia is not a curable disease, but it is treatable. Antipsychotic medications can help treat the positive symptoms associated with the disorder. Psychosocial treatments can address the negative symptoms associated with disorder. In addition, family education, cognitive behavioral therapy, and self-help groups can also help to manage this condition.

Bipolar Disorder

Bipolar disorder describes a disorder that includes alternating episodes of mania (excessive activity, energy, and excitement) and episodes of depression. Bipolar disorder affects approximately 5.7 million adult Americans, or about 2.6% of the U.S. population age 18 and older every year.[1] The median age of onset for bipolar disorder is 25 years, although the illness can start in early childhood or as late as the 40s and 50s.[2] The disorder is found equally in males and females.

This disorder is characterized by dramatic shifts in mood and energy levels. These dramatic fluctuations can affect a person's ability to carry out daily tasks. The shifts in mood and energy levels are more severe than the normal ups and downs that everyone experiences. Manic periods may be characterized by periods of high energy. During these periods, individuals may commit to significant plans, demonstrate pressured speech, and engage in risky behaviors. The behaviors may include financial risks, high spending, or sexually risky activity.

The depressive symptoms may consist of individuals showing low energy with depressive symptoms. These individuals may feel sad, sleep a lot more, feel overwhelmed, or increase eating. The increased eating may consist of specifically increasing carbohydrate intake.

The disorder can be treated with medications including lithium and Abilify®. In addition, counseling can help individuals with symptoms and management. According to the Surgeon General

Report for Mental Health, consumers with bipolar disorder face up to ten years of coping with symptoms before getting an accurate diagnosis, with only one in four receiving an accurate diagnosis in less than three years.

Depressive Disorders

Depressive disorders include disorders that affect how you feel emotionally, such as your level of sadness or happiness. These disorders can disrupt your ability to function. Major depression is one of the most common mental disorders in the United States. Depression is the result of a chemical imbalance, which has been linked to a low level of serotonin. Serotonin is a neurotransmitter in our central nervous system. Researchers have found lower levels of serotonin in the brainstem and cerebrospinal fluid of suicidal individuals. Depression *does* respond to treatment.

Suicide is a potentially preventable public health problem. The National Institute for Mental Health lists suicide as the tenth leading cause of death in the U.S. and estimates there are nearly 40,000 suicides per year. Males are four times more likely to take their lives than females. Suicide has an incredible toll on families and is felt to be preventable. There are usually warning signs that individuals contemplating suicide will exhibit. They are outlined in table 9.1.

TABLE 9.1 WARNING SIGNS FOR SUICIDE

Always talking or thinking about death
Clinical depression, deep sadness, loss of interest, trouble sleeping and eating, that gets worse
Having a "death wish"
Losing interest in things one used to care about
Making comments about being hopeless, helpless, or worthless
Putting affairs in order, tying up loose ends, changing a will
Saying things like "It would be better if I wasn't here" or "I want out"
Sudden, unexpected switch from being very sad to being very calm or appearing to be happy
Talking about suicide or killing one's self

As noted before, depression does respond to treatment. The American College of Physicians (ACP) performed an extensive systematic review of randomized controlled trials that evaluated treatments for depression from 1990 through 2015.[3] Interventions that were evaluated included psychotherapies, ω-3 fatty acids, S-adenosyl-l-methionine, St. John's wort, exercise, and second-generation antidepressants. Following the extensive review, the ACP recommends that clinicians select between either cognitive behavioral therapy or second-generation antidepressants to treat patients with major depressive disorder.

Anxiety Disorders

Anxiety is an emotion characterized by fear. It may involve the anticipation of future misfortune. It is usually characterized as excessive worrying. People with an anxiety disorder may develop avoidance behaviors. Examples of various anxiety disorders include generalized anxiety disorder, panic disorder, and various phobias.

Panic Disorder

Panic disorder, as noted by the National Institute for Mental Health, affects about six million American adults and is twice as common in women than men. Panic attacks typically begin in late adolescent or early adulthood. Genetics is felt to play a role in the development of panic attacks. Individuals experience a feeling of being out of control during a panic attack. These attacks are described as real, fearful episodes. Individuals may begin to develop a worry about the potential for future attacks. This fear may translate into an avoidance of places where panic attacks have occurred in the past.

Physical symptoms are the hallmark of an attack. Individuals will describe a pounding or racing heart, difficulty breathing, sweating, chest or stomach pains, and a feeling of weakness. Repeated panic attacks can lead to a disabling condition of avoidance and even a withdrawal from public places. Some may become housebound due to their fears.

This condition is treatable. Mainstays of treatments include psychotherapy and medications. Psychotherapy will focus on cognitive behavior therapy. This technique will look to teach patients different ways of thinking, behaving, and reacting to situations that help him or her feel less anxious and fearful. Doctors may prescribe medications to help treat panic disorder. The most commonly prescribed medications for panic disorder are anti-anxiety medications and antidepressants.

Trauma- and Stressor-Related Disorders

Trauma and stress disorders are adjustment disorders in which a person has trouble coping during or after a stressful life event. Examples include post-traumatic stress disorder (PTSD) and acute stress disorder.

PTSD

PTSD is a serious condition that can develop after a person has experienced or witnessed a traumatic or terrifying event in which serious physical harm may have occurred or had the potential to occur. PTSD is a lasting consequence of traumatic ordeals that cause intense fear, helplessness, and horror. They can be initiated from a traumatic event involving sexual or physical assault, the unexpected death of a loved one, an accident, war, or a natural disaster.

Symptoms of PTSD include reliving, avoidance behaviors, and increased arousal. "Reliving" is the term that describes the repeated reliving of the traumatic ordeal. It is usually with recurrent thoughts of the ordeal or may involve flashbacks, hallucinations, or nightmares. Avoiding occurs when a patient with PTSD will avoid certain scenarios, people, or places that remind him or her of the trauma. This can lead to isolation. Increased arousal includes excessive emotions, which then lead to relationship difficulties, sleep disturbances, and irritability.

Treatments that are typically utilized include medications and psychotherapies. The serotonin medications used to treat depression can also be used to treat PTSD. Psychotherapies include cognitive behavioral therapies and exposure therapies. Exposure therapies involve having the individual relive the traumatic experience in a controlled setting. Exposure therapy helps the person confront the fear and gradually become more comfortable with situations that were once frightening and anxiety provoking. This has shown to be been very successful at treating PTSD. In addition, family and group therapy have also been shown to be effective in treating PTSD.

CLINICAL PEARL

Research trials are ongoing for a number of mental health disorders. The trials may be evaluating a new medication or counseling intervention. To search for a clinical trial near you, you can visit ClinicalTrials.gov. This is a searchable registry and results database of federally and privately supported clinical trials. The website will give you information about the purpose of the trial, locations, and contact information.

Resources

American Psychiatric Association: Web page for a professional organization of psychiatrists dedicated to promoting mental illness awareness and treatment: https://www.psychiatry.org/

Autism Spectrum Education Network: http://aspennj.org

Austim Speaks: Website that covers all aspects of autism and its impacts; this link reviews Asperger syndrome: https://www.autismspeaks .org/what-autism/asperger-syndrome

National Institutes of Mental Health: Link to the site devoted to mental health topics, specifically schizophrenia: https://www.nimh.nih.gov/ health/topics/schizophrenia/index.shtml

American Board of Professional Psychology: Homepage of the professional psychology board that certifies psychologists: https://www .abpp.org

American Psychological Association: Website of the professional organization that represents psychologists in the U.S.: http://www.apa.org/

Association of State and Provincial Psychology Boards: Site for certification and testing information and oversight of credentials: http://www.asppb.net

Bureau of Labor Statistics: Site that gives an overview of the profession, education, environment, pay, and additional details of the physician-assistant profession: https://www.bls.gov/ooh/life-physical-and-social-science/psychologists.ht

Endnotes

1. Ronald C. Kessler, Wai Tat Chiu, Olga Demler, and Ellen E. Walters, "Prevalence, Severity, and Comorbidity of Twelve-Month DSM-IV Disorders in the National Comorbidity Survey Replication (NCS-R)," *Archives of General Psychiatry* 62, no. 6 (2005): 617–27.
2. Ronald C. Kessler et al., "Lifetime Prevalence and Age-of-Onset Distributions of DSM-IV Disorders in the National Comorbidity Survey Replication (NCS-R)," *Archives of General Psychiatry* 62, no. 6 (2005): 593–602.
3. Amir Qaseem, Michael J. Barry, and Devon Kansagara, "Nonpharmalogic versus Pharmacologic Treatment of Adult Patients With Major Depressive Disorder: A Clinical Practice Guideline From the American College of Physicians," *Annals of Internal Medicine* 164, no. 5 (2016): 350–59, doi:10.7326/M15-2570.

Chapter 10

Marijuana

I have been getting the "Doc should I try medical marijuana?" question with increased regularity among my patients. These patients may include an eighty-year-old woman with chronic nerve pain as well as a forty-year-old male with chronic low back pain. This chapter will review the history of marijuana in the United States and will discuss what we do know in terms of marijuana and its effects on the body, mind, and certain medical conditions.

Recreational Drug Use

"Recreational drug use" is the term used when the drug is used with the primary intention of altering the central nervous system in an attempt for emotional pleasure. The drug may be legal or illegal. Most legal drugs are also controlled substances.

History
Recently, a number of states have legalized the use of marijuana both for medical and recreational purposes. It

may be interesting to know that marijuana was legal in the United States for the first *194 years* of our country's history. Marijuana was recognized for its medicinal uses in the mid-1800s. In fact, cannabis was included in the United States Pharmacopoeia for nearly 100 years.

Most historians feel that the Mexican Revolution was a factor in viewing marijuana negatively. The press described negative concerns over Mexican immigrants and linked these to the use of marijuana, but Congress realized that marijuana held the potential for revenue in the form of taxes. The Marihuana Tax Act of 1937 (Pub. 238, 75th Congress, 50 Stat. 551) was a United States Act that placed a tax on the sale of cannabis.

When the expensive excise tax act did not slow the sale and use of marijuana, political pressure began to increase. Harry J. Anslinger, commissioner of the Federal Bureau of Narcotics, responded to political pressure to ban marijuana at a nationwide level. Congress then passed the Boggs Act of 1952 and the Narcotics Control Act of 1956. These laws lead to mandatory sentencing including both prison time and monetary fines. In *Leary v. United States* (1969), the Supreme Court held the Marihuana Tax Act to be unconstitutional since it violated the Fifth Amendment to the United States Constitution privilege against self-incrimination. In response, Congress passed the Controlled Substances Act as Title II of the Comprehensive Drug Abuse Prevention and Control Act of 1970, which repealed the Marihuana Tax Act.

The Controlled Substances Act defined marijuana as a controlled 1 substance. Controlled 1 substances, as defined by the Drug Enforcement Agency and the Department of Justice, must meet three criteria. First, they are drugs or other substances that have a high potential for abuse. Second, the drug or other substance must have no current accepted medical treatment use in the United States. Lastly, there must be a lack of accepted safety for use of the drug or other substance under medical supervision. The federal government regards marijuana as an illegal substance, but currently permits individual states to regulate its use.

Marijuana

The plant *Cannabis sativa* is the source of marijuana. The active substances in this plant can be found in the leaves, flowers, and stems. The plant contains the mind-altering chemicals known as cannabinoids. Two active cannabinoids include *delta-9-tetrahydrocannabinol* (THC) and cannabidiol (CBD).

Mechanisms of Action

THC acts on specific brain cell receptors. THC is very similar to naturally produced compounds in the body. These compounds play a role in normal brain development and function. Marijuana, and specifically THC, activates different areas of the brain that contain these receptors. Activation of these receptors can cause a variety of responses in the body; each response or action is dependent on the specific region of the brain that is activated. The specific areas of the brain and their functions are outlined in table 10.1.

TABLE 10.1 SPECIFIC BRAIN SITES AFFECTED BY MARIJUANA

Cerebral cortex	Plays a role in memory, thinking, perceptual awareness, and consciousness
Hypothalamus	Governs metabolic processes such as appetite
Brain stem	Controls arousal, vomiting reflex, blood pressure, heart rate, and pain sensation
Hippocampus	Involved in memory storage and recall
Cerebellum	Responsible for coordination and muscle control
Amygdala	Plays a role in emotions

The cerebral cortex is the area of the brain responsible for memory, thinking, and perception. THC can affect this area, leading to alterations in perception that may affect memory. Some individuals have reported that smoking marijuana can lead to the "munchies"; this is due to the interaction of THC on the hypothalamus. The hypothalamus is the area of the brain responsible for appetite and the effect of THC is to increase the appetite drive.

The brain stem is the area of the brain responsible for arousal, blood pressure, heart rate, and nausea/vomiting centers. THC may affect the brain stem by causing an increase in heart rate and the inhibition of nausea/vomiting. It is felt that information from the stomach is communicated to the nucleus of the solitary tract (NTS) in the caudal hindbrain.[1] The hippocampus is the area of the brain involved in memory storage and recall. Marijuana can affect both memory storage and recall, at times invoking vivid flashbacks.

The cerebellum is the area of the brain that is responsible for coordination and muscle control. THC may cause impaired coordination and issues with muscle control. Lastly, there are receptors in the amygdala that are affected by marijuana. The amygdala is the area of the brain that plays a role in emotions. The effects of marijuana may impact certain emotions. Cannabis has been shown to affect users' ability to recognize, process, and empathize with human emotions like happiness, sadness, and anger.[2]

Cognitive Effects

Marijuana also affects brain development. When marijuana users begin using as teenagers, the drug may reduce thinking, memory, and learning functions. It may also affect how the brain builds connections between regions of the brain necessary for these functions. One study showed that people aged 13 to 38 who started smoking marijuana heavily in their teens and had an ongoing cannabis use disorder lost an average of eight IQ points. The diminished mental abilities did not fully return in those individuals who quit marijuana as adults. Those who started smoking marijuana as adults did not show notable IQ declines.[3] Multiple sclerosis (MS) is a neurological disease that may cause painful muscles spasms. Research has shown that muscle spasms may be reduced with marijuana use. However, MS is also associated with cognitive (thinking) difficulties. A well-controlled study determined that patients with MS who smoke cannabis are more cognitively impaired than nonusers.[4]

Positive Effects

The National Institute of Health (NIH) has supported cannabis research to determine its potential positive effects on certain conditions and diseases. Since marijuana was illegal in the United States for an extended period, most medical claims were anecdotal. Recently, medical effects of marijuana are being evaluated in clinical trials.

There is growing interest in the marijuana chemical *cannabidiol* (CBD) to treat certain conditions such as childhood epilepsy, a disorder that causes a child to seizure. Therefore, scientists have been specially breeding marijuana plants and making CBD in an oil form for treatment purposes. In addition, CBD is a cannabinoid that does not affect the mind or adversely affect behavior. The NIH feels it may be useful for reducing pain and inflammation, controlling epileptic seizures, and possibly even treating mental illness and addictions. However, there is no current approved medical use for marijuana to treat mental illness.

One recent animal study has shown that marijuana extracts may help kill certain types of cancer cells and reduce the size of others. Evidence from one cell culture study suggests that purified extracts from whole-plant marijuana can slow the growth of cancer cells from one of the most serious types of brain tumors. Research in mice showed that treatment with purified extracts of THC and CBD when used with radiation increased the cancer-killing effects of the radiation.[5] Research has not shown this to be true for humans at this time.

Glaucoma is a condition in which there is an abnormal buildup of intraocular (meaning within the eye) pressure (IOP); if left untreated it can lead to blindness. Research has found that smoking marijuana will lower IOP. However, according to the American Academy of Ophthalmology the IOP is only lowered for a short period of time, about three or four hours. Since the IOP needs to be lowered at all times, marijuana use would not provide the necessary coverage to treat this disease.

Currently, there are two cannabinoids (dronabinol and nabilone) approved by the U.S. Food and Drug Administration (FDA) that prevent or treat chemotherapy-related nausea and vomiting.

Negative Effects

Much like all medications, even though there are positive effects, there are also side effects or potential negative effects. We know that marijuana can be addictive. Research suggests that about 1 in 11 users becomes addicted to marijuana and will seek it out on a daily or more frequent basis.[6]

Users also report less academic and career success. For example, marijuana use is linked to a higher likelihood of dropping out of school.[7] In addition, marijuana use has also been shown to lead to more job absences, accidents, and injuries.[8]

Marijuana smokers can develop a lung infection from a mold called aspergillosis. Aspergillus is a mold that is found on marijuana leaves. The mold may be inhaled when the marijuana leaves are smoked and inhaled. Some infections caused by mold are known as opportunistic infections, meaning they will infect susceptible individuals. Typically, these susceptible individuals have a weakened immune system. Immune systems are weakened in organ transplant patients, patients with AIDS, or patients recently receiving chemotherapy. In addition, medications used to treat inflammatory arthritis (rheumatoid or psoriatic) may also weaken the immune system. Aspergillus can cause an infection in the lung (pneumonia) and even death. The American Thoracic Society does not recommend smoking marijuana in individuals with a compromised immune system.

Potpourri

As previously noted, more effects of marijuana use will be studied in the future. The National Academics of Sciences in January of 2017 produced a paper detailing what we currently know regarding the use of marijuana. The findings are summarized in table 10.2. The use of the drug will continue to provoke debates regarding both the positive and negative effects associated with its use.

TABLE 10.2 SUMMARY OF CURRENT RESEARCH REGARDING MARIJUANA USE

- MS-related muscle spasms and chemotherapy-induced nausea and vomiting are responsive to oral cannabinoids
- Use increases risk of being in a motor vehicle accident (MVA)
- Use does not increase of risk of lung, head, and neck cancers
- Evidence suggests that cannabis smoking may trigger a heart attack
- Use is associated with more frequent bronchitis episodes; unclear if use increases other respiratory diseases
- Use is associated with an increased risk of developing schizophrenia
- Moderate evidence suggests that use leads to increased tobacco, alcohol, and other illicit drugs
- Learning, memory, and attention are impaired right after use

The National Academics of Sciences January 12, 2017

CLINICAL PEARL

Legalization of marijuana is approved by a number of states for both medical and recreational usage. The benefits to the individualized states are obvious regarding taxation benefits. The federal government also sees financial benefits in indirect ways.

A recent study examined all prescriptions filled by Medicare Part D (see chapter 12 for additional information) for enrollees between 2010–2013 in 17 states and Washington DC where marijuana is legalized. In these states, prescription drug use fell by 0.5% with an estimated savings of $165 million in 2013 alone.[9] If the numbers are extrapolated it is estimated that $470 million may be saved by Medicare Part D if approved by all 50 states.

Resources

MedlinePlus: Web page that updates medical uses for marijuana: https://medlineplus.gov/ency/patientinstructions/000899.htm

National Cancer Institute: Web page that updates the latest possible uses of marijuana for cancer treatments: https://www.cancer.gov/about-cancer/treatment/cam/patient/cannabis-pdq

American Academy of Ophthalmology: https://www.aao.org/

American Thoracic Society, Patient Education: http://www.thoracic.org/patients/patient-resources/resources/marijuana.pdf

Endnotes

1. Charles C. Horn, "Why Is the Neurobiology of Nausea and Vomiting so Important?" *Appetite* 50, nos. 2–3 (2008): 430–434. doi:10.1016/j.appet.2007.09.015.

2. Lucy J. Troup et al., "An Event-Related Potential Study on the Effects of Cannabis on Emotion Processing," *PLoS ONE* 11, no. (2016): e0149764, doi:10.1371/journal.pone.0149764

3. Madeline H. Meier et al., "Persistent Cannabis Users Show Neuropsychological Decline from Childhood to Midlife," *Proceedings of the National Academy of Sciences USA* 109, no. (2012): E2657–E2664.

4. Bennis Pavisian et al., "Effects of Cannabis on Cognition in Patients with MS: A Psychometric and MRI Study," *Neurology* 82, no. 21 (2014): 1879–1887, doi:10.1212/WNL.0000000000000446

5. Katherine A. Scott, Angus G. Dalgleish, and Wai M. Liu, "The Combination of Cannabidiol and Δ9-Tetrahydrocannabinol Enhances the Anticancer Effects of Radiation in an Orthotopic Murine Glioma Model," *Molecular Cancer Therapeutics* 13, no. (2014): 2955–67.

6. James C. Anthony, Lynn A. Warner, and Ronald C. Kessler, "Comparative Epidemiology of Dependence on Tobacco, Alcohol, Controlled Substances, and Inhalants: Basic Findings from the National Comorbidity Survey," *Experimental and Clinical Psychopharmacology* 2, no. 3 (1994): 244–68; Rosalie Liccardo Pacula and Wayne Denis Hall, *Cannabis Use and*

Dependence: Public Health and Public Policy (Cambridge, UK: Cambridge University Press, 2003).

7. Daniel F. McCaffrey, Rosalie Liccardo Pacula, Bing Han, and Phyllis Ellickson, "Marijuana Use and High School Dropout: The Influence of Unobservables." *Health Economics* 19, no. 11 (2010): 1281–1299.

8. Craig Zwerling, James Ryan, and Endel John Orav, "The Efficacy of Preemployment Drug Screening for Marijuana and Cocaine in Predicting Employment Outcome," *JAMA* 264, no. 20 (199): 2639–2643.

9. Ashley C. Bradford and W. David Bradford, "Medical Marijuana Laws Reduce Prescription Medication Use in Medicare part D," *Health Affairs* 35, no. 7 (2016): 1230–36.

Chapter 11

Sexual Health

S ex. The term evokes a myriad of images and reactions. This chapter will discuss the health issues associated with sex and more specifically focus on the diseases that are transmitted through sexual activity. It is important to have a basic understanding of the different sexually transmitted diseases (STDs) and sexually transmitted infections (STIs) and their potential immediate and long-term effects on the body. The latter portion of the chapter will discuss the various testing options for STD/STIs.

Conditions

The term *curable* applies to a disease or sickness that can be treated with either a drug or proper medicine and the problem will be resolved. *Treatable* is the medical term that indicates a disease or sickness is capable of being improved with a medicine or treatment. Treatable and curable are different terms.

Latex Condoms

Latex condoms are used to cover the penis and prevent the spread of semen, which contains sperm, from entering the female reproductive tract. The CDC reports that when latex condoms are used every time and put on early enough and correctly, they reduce chances of pregnancy over a one-year period to 3 percent, compared to 85 percent without their use. Likewise, condoms cut the risk of human immunodeficiency virus (HIV) infection per year from about 80 percent to less than a 1 percent chance of infection.

Condoms act as a barrier to prevent blood, semen, or vaginal fluids from passing from one person to the other during intercourse. Some diseases that are transmitted sexually are present in the semen, blood, or vaginal fluids and can pass from an infected individual to their sexual partner. Condoms are made of latex (rubber) or polyurethane for individuals allergic to latex. The CDC warns that the package of the condom should state that the condoms have been shown to prevent disease. This statement means the condom has passed a quality-control process. The condoms are filled with water and checked for leaks. An average of 996 of 1,000 condoms must pass this test to meet quality-control standards. It should be noted, given this method of testing that four out of one thousand condoms may not provide complete barrier protection.

Gonorrhea

Gonorrhea is an STD that is caused by the bacteria *Neisseria gonorrhoeae*. Gonorrhea is both treatable and curable. The risks of acquiring gonorrhea from an infected partner as estimated by the CDC is 20 percent in males and 50 percent in females.

Symptoms associated with gonorrhea infection can affect multiple sites in the body. The rectum may be involved, especially in cases of anal sex involving penile-rectum penetration. Rectal infection may manifest with discharge from the rectum, bleeding, and anal itching. The eyes may also be involved and develop an infection with associated discharge. Gonorrhea can lead to photophobia (sensitivity to light), pain, and eye drainage. The joints of the body may also become infected, a condition that is not only very painful but also a medical emergency. Joint infection, also known as septic arthritis, requires immediate antibiotics and possible drainage of the infected joints.

In males, symptoms from gonorrhea infection may only be apparent *10 percent* of the time. If symptoms are present, dysuria (pain when urinating) will be very common. Penile discharge may also be present; the color of the discharge can range from white to yellow to green. Less commonly, the testicles may be swollen or tender.

Gonorrhea symptoms in females are present only about *30 percent* of the time, so most women will not have obvious symptoms. The concern is that if the infection is left untreated, more serious complications will arise. These symptoms include dysuria (painful urination), vaginal discharge, and vaginal bleeding outside of normal menses.

The diagnosis of gonorrhea can be done by swabbing the endocervical region in women or urethral region in men. Alternatively, a blood test can also be performed to confirm the diagnosis. If the diagnosis is confirmed, then it is important to contact previous sex partners from the past two months so they can be tested and receive possible treatment. Treatment is done with antibiotics. The recommended antibiotics are ceftriaxone, given as a single intramuscular injection, or azithromycin taken by mouth in a single dose.

If gonorrhea is left untreated in the female, pelvic inflammatory disease (PID) can occur. The gonorrhea infection can lead to collections of infected fluid (abscesses) to develop in the fallopian tubes. These are the tubes that connect the ovaries to the uterus. The ovaries release eggs for fertilization, which travel to the fallopian tubes and if fertilized will implant in the uterus. Gonorrhea and other infections can cause scar tissue, produce abscesses, and damage to the reproductive organs. Complications may include infertility, chronic pain, and ectopic pregnancy. PID and repeated infections can increase the risk of infertility. The infections have a cumulative effect on infertility. PID is associated with chronic lower abdominal or pelvic pain. PID may also cause dyspareunia (pain during intercourse). Ectopic pregnancy refers to a fertilized egg not implanting normally in the uterus but in the fallopian tube. The failure to implant in the uterus may be due to a blockage of the fallopian tube. Ectopic pregnancies can be life-threatening emergencies that may require emergency.

Doctors diagnose PID based on signs and symptoms of the patient. They may also perform a pelvic examination. Diagnostic testing will also include an analysis of vaginal discharge and cervical cultures. Testing of the urine may also be done to test for a urinary tract infection (bladder infection). Treatment for PID includes a course of antibiotics for both the patient and his or her partner and a period of abstinence to prevent reinfection.

Chlamydia

Chlamydia is an infection caused by the bacteria *Chlamydia trachomatis*. Chlamydia is both treatable and curable. It is caused by an infection of the cervix (cervicitis) in women. Men may get infections of the urethra (urethritis) or rectum (proctitis). The CDC notes that chlamydia is the most frequently reported bacterial sexually transmitted infection in the United States. In 2014, 1,441,789 cases of chlamydia were reported to the CDC, but an estimated 2.86 million infections occur annually. Chlamydia is most common among young people. Almost two thirds of new chlamydia infections occur among youth aged 15–24 years. The CDC also estimates that one in twenty sexually active young women aged 14–24 years have chlamydia.

Chlamydia infections commonly involve the cervix, urethra, and eye(s). The infection is diagnosed by a vaginal swab in women and a urine specimen for men. The urine specimen may also be an alternative method for testing in women. The treatment for infection is the same as the treatment for gonorrhea. The two bacteria are commonly found together. Doxycycline is used for bacterial resistant cases and should be taken twice a day for ten days.

HPV

While chlamydia is the most common bacterial infection, HPV is the most common sexually transmitted infection (STI). It is caused by a virus. HPV is treatable but not curable. It is also potentially preventable, with vaccination. The virus will characteristically cause warts in the genital area. The genital warts usually appear as a small bump or group of bumps. They can range in size from small to large and can be flat, raised, or cauliflower in shape.

Diagnosis is typically made by a health care provider by visual examination of the warts. The warts can be treated. If the genital warts are left untreated, sometimes they will resolve on their own; they may stay the same or grow both in size and number. They are treated with a variety of options. Creams such as podofilox and imiquimod can be prescribed by a health care provider. They are applied intermittently to warts for a period of up to four weeks. The warts may also be frozen off with liquid nitrogen, surgically resected, treated with electrocautery (application of an electric current), or removed with use of a laser.

The warts may be unsightly and embarrassing. It is important to remember that the types of HPV that can cause genital warts are not the same as the types of HPV that can cause cancers. The high-risk types HPV 16 and 18 are responsible for approximately 70 percent of cervical cancers.[1] The low-risk non-oncogenic HPV types include HPV 6 and 11 cause anogenital warts and recurrent respiratory papillomatosis.[2]

The concern with HPV is that it can lead to cancer. Cervical cancer is the most common cancer, but HPV can also cause cancer of the vulva, vagina, penis, or anus. It is for this reason that it is recommended sexually active females be evaluated by health care providers on an annual basis. The doctor may take swab cells of the cervix to evaluate for the presence of HPV. If HPV—specifically, the subtypes associated with cancer—is found, then regular evaluation of the cervix and an annual PAP test should be done. The surface of the cervix may also be viewed using a special magnifying device, the colposcope in order to perform a colposcopy. This procedure looks closely for abnormal changes on the surface of the cervix, vagina, and vulva. These types of cancers often take years to develop.

The CDC reports, among women diagnosed with an HPV cancer, cervical cancer is the most common, with about eleven thousand women diagnosed annually in the United States; subsequently about 4,400 women die every year from cervical cancer in our country. For men in the United States diagnosed with an HPV cancer, oropharyngeal cancer is the most common. Around 7,200 U.S. men each year are diagnosed with oropharyngeal cancer caused by HPV infection.

HPV infection may be preventable. HPV vaccines are available and are now routinely recommended for 11- and 12-year-old girls and boys. Vaccination is also recommended for females ages 13 through 26 years and males ages 13 through 21 years who were not vaccinated when they were younger. The CDC also recommends a vaccination for men who have sex with men and men aged 22 through 26 years who were not vaccinated when they were younger. The quadrivalent vaccine is directed against HPV 6, 11, 16, and 18; the bivalent vaccine is directed against HPV 16 and 18. The HPV vaccines are given in three shots over six months; as with any vaccination, it is important to get all three doses, as this will increase the chances of an effective response.

Research has evaluated the effectiveness of the HPV vaccines and found the vaccine efficacy against lesions related to the specific HPV types to be 96 percent for cervical cancer, 100 percent for both vulvar and vaginal cancers, and 99 percent for genital warts. Vaccine efficacy against any lesion (regardless of HPV type) for cervical cancers was 30 percent.[3]

Genital Herpes

Genital herpes has historically been caused by the HSV-2 virus. Genital herpes is treatable but not curable. The CDC estimates that in the United States about one out of every six people aged 14 to 49 years have genital herpes. It is also estimated that 776,000 people in the United States get new herpes infections every year. Nationwide,

15.5 percent of persons aged 14 to 49 years have HSV-2 infection, and 80 percent don't know they have it. There is no cure for herpes. However, there are medicines that can treat, prevent, or shorten outbreaks.

Infections are transmitted through contact with lesions, genital secretions, or oral secretions. HSV-1 and HSV-2 can also be shed from skin that looks normal. Generally, a person can only get an HSV-2 infection during sexual contact with someone who has a genital HSV-2 infection. Transmission most commonly occurs from an infected partner who may *not* have visible lesions or sores and commonly may not know he or she is infected.

Genital herpes may be characterized by fluid-filled blisters on the genitals. Condoms do not provide reliable protection, as the virus is spread when it touches another person's skin. You can *contract* the virus even if there are *no active blisters* on the genitals. One study found that in 70 percent of patients, transmission appeared to result from sexual contact during periods of asymptomatic viral shedding (without obvious lesions).[4] Both early and late lesions can occur with herpes.

Treatment for genital herpes is done during symptomatic eruptions. The eruptions are more likely to occur during times of stress. On average, there are typically four to six flares per year. The flares are treated with antiviral medications. Valcyclovir or acyclovir are typically used to shorten the length of the flare.

HIV

HIV is a virus that is sexually transmitted. HIV is treatable but not curable. HIV was first reported in the 1980s. The virus attacks white blood cells, specifically the T cells. These are the cells that the body uses to fight infections and to provide surveillance against potential cancers. The diagnosis of HIV is done with a blood test. The test will look for specific antibodies that the body uses to fight the virus. It may take the body anywhere from six weeks to one year to develop the antibodies, thus producing a positive test result may take time. Follow-up tests may be needed, depending on the initial time of exposure.

Early testing is crucial, as it permits early identification and early treatment. Treatments consist of a cocktail of medications that are known as combination antiretroviral therapy (ART). These medications will attack the human immunodeficiency virus at multiple stages of its life cycle. The medications of today are life saving and life sustaining. Today a 20-year-old HIV-positive adult on ART in the United States or Canada is expected to live into his or her early 70s, a life expectancy approaching that of the general population.[5]

Syphilis

Syphilis is an STD that is caused by the bacteria *Treponema pallidum*. Syphilis is treatable and curable. The CDC estimates that in 2014 that there were 63,450 reported new cases of syphilis. The syphilis rate is increasing among the male homosexual population. This group accounted for 83 percent of all new cases reported. Syphilis can be transmitted from person to person via direct contact with a syphilitic sore. The sore is known as a chancre. Chancres occur mainly on the external genitals, vagina, anus, or rectum. They can also occur on the lips and in the mouth. Their location is dependent on the type of sex being performed.

Transmission of syphilis occurs during vaginal, anal, or oral sex. Pregnant women with this disease may transmit it to their unborn child. Syphilis can be cured with the right antibiotics from a health care provider. However, treatment will not undo any damage that the infection has already done. Previous or past infection does not prevent future infection. Long-term complications can occur if not treated correctly.

Symptoms in adults are divided into stages: primary, secondary, or latent. The primary stage may be characterized by a single sore or multiple sores or chancres. The sore is located where syphilis entered the body. The sore is usually firm, round, and painless. The sore lasts three to six weeks and heals regardless of whether the person receives treatment. Even though the sore recedes with time, individuals must still receive treatment so the infection does not move to the secondary stage.

During the secondary stage, patients may have skin rashes and/or sores in the mouth, vagina, or anus (also called mucous membrane lesions). This stage usually starts with a rash on one or more areas of the body. The rash can show up when the primary sore is healing or several weeks after the sore has healed. The rash can look like rough, red, or reddish-brown spots on the palms of the hands and/or the bottoms of the feet. The rash is not itchy. The symptoms from this stage will go away whether or not you receive treatment. Without treatment, the infection will progress to the latent stage of syphilis.

The latent stage of syphilis may begin after individuals have had syphilis for years and without active signs or symptoms. Most people with untreated syphilis do not develop latent stage syphilis. Symptoms of the late stage of syphilis include difficulty coordinating your muscle movements, paralysis (not able to move certain parts of your body), numbness, blindness, and dementia (mental disorder with an inability to remember). There is also the potential for damage to internal organs or even death.

Diagnosis and Testing

Getting tested for a STD/STI can feel awkward, and many patients may be uncomfortable discussing their concerns with their physician. This should not be the case; remember most physicians have seen and heard it all. Some patients may feel comfortable bringing up their concerns of an STI to their primary care physician, while others may not. Physicians who regularly treat STIs include gynecologists and urologists. Dermatologists also treat STIs if seeing skin lesions related to the infection. Advantages of seeing a physician for testing and treatment include your health insurance covering the services, physician's knowledge of your past medical history/current medications, and convenience of being seen in the office. Other options for testing include an STD clinic, online testing, and home kits.

Testing at a STD clinic is another option for consumers. Locating a clinic can be done easily at the website https://gettested.cdc.gov/Testing; just enter your zip code and you will be provided with a list of clinics. Testing at a clinic has a number of advantages: access to a wider range of tests, (including rapid testing, which can provide instant results), clinicians who stay up to date on the latest treatments, and reduced testing costs. Disadvantages can include limited hours and feeling uncomfortable visiting an STD clinic. Online STD testing allows consumers to purchase tests online, receive a prescription for specific tests, and then report to testing centers to provide urine or blood samples.

When to get tested is not always a straightforward answer, since a great deal of STIs can be asymptomatic. Testing and evaluation is recommended for any new skin lesion of the genital/oral/anal areas, new onset of painful urination, or pain with intercourse. Some patients also wish to get screened on a regular basis, upon starting a new sexual relationship, having a history of multiple partners, or being made aware of an unfaithful partner. If there is a concern for a STI/STD, it is probably best to get screened to remove any anxiety or potential concern.

CLINICAL PEARL

Less Risky Sex Versus Safe Sex

Marketing campaigns have advocated using condoms for safe sex. Safe implies it is without risk. It is important to know, however, that condoms cannot completely protect you and your partner from some STDs. According to the National Institutes of Health, condoms are impervious to the smallest viruses. Condoms, however, can break or slip off 1 percent to 2 percent of the time. The use of petroleum-based products (such as Vaseline) for lubrication can cause breakdown of the latex condom. Additionally, surveys show most people do not use condoms properly or consistently, and roughly 12 million Americans each year contract an STD.

Individual studies have shown that the transmission rates for various STDs differ greatly. None of the transmission rates drop to 0 percent with the use of condoms. One study examined the transmission rate for women in acquiring gonorrhea and chlamydia from infected males and showed the use of condoms will produce a 62 percent reduced risk of acquiring gonorrhea and a 26 percent reduction in the risk of acquiring chlamydial infection.[6] Another study followed adolescent African American females and combined incidence of gonorrhea, chlamydial infection, or trichomoniasis and found the girls who reported using condoms developed at least one STD at a rate of 17.8 percent compared with a rate of 30 percent in the girls who did not report using condoms consistently.[7] The effectiveness of condoms in protecting against HPV infection and HPV-related conditions such as genital warts and cervical cancer has also been evaluated. A meta-analysis of 20 studies found no evidence that condoms were effective against a genital HPV infection.[8] Another study followed 444 female college students looking at the incidence of genital HPV infection. The study found that consistently using condoms with a new partner was not associated with significant protection against HPV.[9] HIV transmission rates with condom use have also been studied. It is thought that condom use will reduce the risk of transmission of HIV by 80 percent, with a range of 35 percent to 94 percent.[10] The difference in protection rates may be related to the specific type of STD tested. Some are viral in origin, and others are bacterial. For HPV, intimate contact prior to sexual intercourse may allow for spread of the virus to the hands and then to the genitals. Similar transmission may occur with gonorrhea and chlamydia since both are from bacteria.

It is important to remember that if you develop symptoms previously discussed in this chapter and consistently use condoms, you are still at risk for an STD. Regular—and as needed—evaluation by your physician to address concerns and to avoid long-term complications of STDs is recommended.

Endnotes

1. Silvia de Sanjose et al., "Human Papillomavirus Genotype Attribution in Invasive Cervical Cancer: A Retrospective Cross-Sectional Worldwide Study," *Lancet Oncology* 11, no. 11 (2010): 1048–1056.

2. Charles J. N. Lacey, Catherine M. Lowndes, and Keerti V. Shah, "Burden and Management of Non-Cancerous HPV-Related Conditions: HPV-6/11 Disease," *Vaccine* 24, no. S3 (2006): 35–41.

3. FUTURE I/II Study Group, "Four-Year Efficacy of Prophylactic Human Papillomavirus Quadrivalent Vaccine against Low-Grade Cervical, Vulvar, and Vaginal Intraepithelial Neoplasia and Anogenital Warts: Randomised Controlled Trial," *BMJ* 341 (2010): c3493, doi:10.1136/bmj.c3493.

4. Gregory J. Mertz et al., "Risk Factors for the Sexual Transmission of Genital Herpes," *Annals of Internal Medicine* 116, no. 3 (1992): 197–202.

5. Jorge Sanchez et al., "Prevention of Sexually Transmitted Diseases (STDs) in Female Sex Workers: Prospective Evaluation of Condom Promotion and Strengthened STD Services," *Sexually Transmitted Diseases* 30 (2003): 273–279.

6. Hasina Samji et al., "Closing the Gap: Increases in Life Expectancy among Treated HIV-Positive Individuals in the United States and Canada," *PLoS ONE* 8, no. 12 (2013): e81355. doi:10.1371/journal.pone.0081355.

7. Richard A. Crosby et al., "Value of Consistent Condom Use: A Study of Sexually Transmitted Disease Prevention among African American Adolescent Females," *American Journal of Public Health* 93 (2003): 901–902.

8. Lisa E. Manhart and Laura A. Koutsky, "Do Condoms Prevent Genital HPV Infection, External Genital Warts, or Cervical Neoplasia? A meta-analysis," *Sexually Transmitted Diseases* 29 (2002): 725–735.

9. Rachel L. Winer et al., "Genital Human Papillomavirus Infection: Incidence and Risk Factors in a Cohort of Female University Students. *American Journal of Epidemiology* 157, no. 3 (2003): 218–226.

10. Susan C. Weller and Karen Davis-Beaty, "Condom Effectiveness in Reducing Heterosexual HIV Transmission," *Cochrane Library*, no. 4 (2007).

Chapter 12

Insurance

P atients often tell me that they have "good insurance." I would agree that most consumers feel they have good insurance until the time comes when they have to use it. Many consumers will get an unpleasant realization after receiving a medical bill and see how little the insurance actually paid for the services billed. This chapter will focus on learning the necessary terms associated with insurance plans. It is not only vital to know what the various insurance terms mean, but also to understand how they will affect both you and your family. This chapter will also list the different insurance products that are available.

Premium
Premium is the monthly fee that is paid to a health plan/ insurance company for health coverage. The lower the premium the less money you will need to pay for coverage. The premiums charged by insurance companies or by health plans continue to increase yearly at a rate that exceeds the annual inflation rate.

Deductible

Deductible is the term used to describe the amount you will need to pay out of your pocket before your health insurance plan begins to pay for medical care you received. Therefore, it is in your best financial interest to have low deductibles. For example, if your deductible is $1,500, you will need to spend $1,500 before your insurance plan will begin to cover any medical costs.

Coinsurance

Coinsurance refers to your share of the costs of a covered health care service and usually occurs *after* the entire deductible has paid or met by the consumer. Coinsurance can be calculated as a percentage (for example, 20 percent) of the allowed amount for the service. For example, if the health insurance plan allowed amount for an office visit is $100 and you have met your deductible, your 20 percent coinsurance payment would be $20. The health insurance company will pay the rest.

Allowed Amount

Allowed amount is the maximum amount that payment will be covered by health care services. This term may appear on your healthcare summary or on your bill. Allowed amount may also be called "eligible expense," "payment allowance," or "negotiated rate." If your healthcare provider charges more than the allowed amount, you may be responsible to pay the difference.

Copayment

Copayment is a fixed amount you pay for a covered health care service, usually after you receive the service. The copayment amount can vary by your particular insurance plan as well as the service provided. Your insurance card may list copayment amounts on the card. The amounts owed will vary according to the service provided and may include an office visit to a primary care provider, an office visit to a specialist, an emergency room visit, preventive services, and mental health services.

Flexible Spending Account (FSA)

FSA is an arrangement you set up through your employer to pay for your out-of-pocket medical expenses. These expenses include insurance copayments, deductibles, qualified prescription drugs, and medical devices. The advantage of such a plan is that money for these services is put into an account before taxes. Consumers do not have to pay taxes on any money placed into an FSA. The employer's plan will set a limit on the amount you can put into an FSA each year. One disadvantage to the FSA is that there is no carryover of FSA funds year to year. Some plans may have a $2^{1}/_{2}$-month grace period after the end of the FSA year. The FSA plan can be helpful for individuals with fairly fixed and predictable medical costs over a 12-month period. For example, if they have $400 in fixed medical costs per month, they will put $4,800 into an FSA. If they are in the 18 percent income tax bracket they will thus save 18 percent of $4,800 or $864 in one year.

Health Savings Accounts (HSAs)

HSAs were created in 2003 for individuals with high-deductible health plans to save money for medical expenses. The money placed into an HSA is similar to FSA in that it is tax free. Unlike FSAs the HSA plan is individually owned and is not affected if you change jobs. One can deposit money into his or her HSA, where it earns interest tax free. Funds are not taxed when they are used for qualified medical expenses. The federal government sets annual limits for HSAs. In 2018, the limits were $3,450 for individuals and $6,900 for family. The deadline for contributions to the HSA is the same as an individual retirement account (IRA), April 15 of the following year.

Insurance Products

There are different insurance products that are available to provide medical coverage. Medicare and Medicaid are government-sponsored plans for the elderly, disabled, or poor. Private insurance plans provide additional options for insurance.

Medicare

The idea of a federally funded insurance program had been discussed for a few decades. President Lyndon B. Johnson's goal was to begin a federally funded insurance program for the elderly in America. He envisioned the program as one that provides low-cost medical and hospital care for the elderly. According to the LBJ Presidential Library, before Medicare half of the country's population over age 65 had no medical insurance, and a third of the elderly lived in poverty, unable to afford proper medical care. President Johnson signed Medicare into law on July 30, 1965. President Johnson credited President Truman with originating the idea during his presidency decades before and awarded the first two Medicare cards to President Truman and his wife.

Over the years, Congress has made changes to Medicare. The changes have expanded the coverage, allowing more people to become eligible. In 1972, Medicare was expanded to cover the disabled, people with end-stage renal disease (ESRD) requiring dialysis or kidney transplant, and people 65 or older who select Medicare coverage. Children's Health Insurance Program (CHIP) was created in 1997. The intent of the program was to cover uninsured children. The Medicare Prescription Drug Improvement and Modernization Act of 2003 (MMA) made the biggest changes to the Medicare in the program in 38 years. The MMA created and acknowledged private health plans known as Medicare Advantage Plans. These plans are referred to as Medicare Part C. The MMA also expanded Medicare to include an optional prescription drug benefit. This went into effect in 2006 and is known as Medicare Part D.

The Patient Protection and Affordable Care Act (PPACA), commonly called the Affordable Care Act (ACA), also referred to as Obamacare, was signed into law by President Barack Obama in 2010. It represented the most significant changes to Medicare and Medicaid Act since its inception in 1965. The ACA created the health insurance marketplace, a single place where consumers can apply for and enroll in private health insurance plans. It also expanded Medicaid coverage by raising the minimum income levels to qualify for the programs for both individuals and families. The ACA eliminated the insurer's ability to discriminate or deny insurance based upon pre-existing medical conditions. It also allowed for children to be covered on their parent's insurance plans until the age of 26 years old. Additional provisions of the act focused on tax penalties for the uninsured.

Medicare Part A

Medicare Part A is hospital insurance. Part A covers inpatient care provided in hospitals as well as skilled nursing facilities. It also helps cover hospice care and some at-home health care. Beneficiaries must meet certain conditions to get these benefits. There is typically no monthly premium required for Medicare Part A, provided that either you or your spouse paid Medicare taxes while working. Part A is largely funded by revenue from a 2.9 percent payroll tax levied on employers and workers (each pay 1.45 percent).

Medicare pays hospitals and healthcare systems using a prospective payment system. This system provides the health care institution with a set amount of money that is used for the care provided to the patient. The amount of money is a fixed amount based on the condition and not based on the actual amount of care provided to the patient. The hospital can make money if it spends fewer resources (less tests, shorter length of stay) and conversely lose money if it spends more resources on the patient. The payment to the hospital is based on a diagnosis-related group (DRG), the diagnosis the patient is admitted to at the hospital. To keep the system in check and to prevent substandard care and premature discharges, Medicare penalizes hospitals for readmissions.

Medicare Part B

Part B is medical insurance that helps to cover physician's services and outpatient care. It also covers some other medical services, such as the services of physical and occupational therapists and some at-home health care. It also covers the cost of supplies (durable medical equipment) when it is medically necessary. Part B premium varies by income, with the minimum contribution being $104.90 each month.

Medicare Part C

Medicare Part C is also known as the Medicare *advantage plan.* After the passage of the Balanced Budget Act of 1997, Medicare beneficiaries were allowed to either receive their original Medicare benefits through capitated health insurance Part C plans, or through the original fee-for-service Medicare payment system. The premiums vary by plan. If the Medicare beneficiary chooses the Medicare C option, then he or she does not have the traditional Part A and Part B. His or her Medicare C plan covers both Part A and Part B costs and services. There are a number of factors to consider when choosing a Medicare advantage plan. Some plans may offer gym or health club memberships, prescription plans or lower premiums. It is important to remember that the Medicare advantage plan may have a smaller network and may lack a nationwide network.

There are some publications including *U.S. News and World Report* that rank the plans and other sites that can help to determine which plan may be the best for an individual to choose. The choice should be based on both current and anticipated medical needs.

Medicare Part D

Prescription drug coverage is provided under Medicare Part D. This part was added due to the increasing costs of prescription medications. Medicare Part D is available to everyone with Medicare. This coverage is to help lower prescription drug costs and to protect against higher costs in the future. People will pay a monthly premium for this coverage. The monthly premiums are based on income.

Medicare Supplemental Insurance

Medigap plans are private health insurance plans sold to supplement Medicare. Medigap insurance provides coverage for the copays and some of the co-insurance related costs of the traditional Medicare plan. The name is derived from the notion that it exists to cover the difference or "gap" between the expenses reimbursed to providers by Medicare Parts A and B. The Medigap plans are available to participants in Medicare Parts A and B. Participants in Medicare Part C or the Medicare advantage plans are not eligible for the Medigap plan. The Medicare website can be a very valuable resource in determining which plan may be offered in your area. The website will also list which of the various plans cover hospice care, foreign travel, blood, skilled nursing services, and out-of-pocket limits. The choice of obtaining a Medigap plan as well as choosing the specific Medigap plan should be based on one's current and anticipated medical needs.

Medicaid

When Medicaid was enacted into law in 1965, it provided medical insurance to people receiving cash assistance or the very poor. The program has been expanded over the years. Today a much larger group is covered: low-income families, pregnant women, individuals with disabilities, and people who require long-term care. Children are also covered under the children's insurance program (CHIP). According to the Medicaid website, this program covers roughly 23 percent of the American population. Medicaid is a hybrid of a federal-state program. The federal government sets minimum guidelines for Medicaid eligibility, but states can choose to expand coverage beyond the minimum threshold. The states can adjust the programs to best serve the people in their state. For this reason, there is a wide variation in the services offered from state to state.

Health Maintenance Organization (HMO)

A health maintenance organization (HMO) is a type of health insurance plan that usually *limits* coverage to care from doctors who work for or who are contracted with the HMO. It generally will not cover out-of-network care except in the case of an emergency. An HMO may require you to live or work in its service area to be eligible for coverage. HMOs often provide integrated care and focus on prevention and wellness. HMO plans tend to have very low premiums and lower deductibles. It does require the insured to obtain a primary care physician (PCP). The plan will usually require one to get a referral from their PCP to see a specialist. For this reason, the PCP may be referred to as a gate keeper. These plans may have a very limited network and may not cover out-of-network services.

Preferred Provider Organization (PPO)

A preferred provider organization (PPO) is a health plan that contracts with medical providers, such as hospitals and doctors, to create a network of participating providers. You pay less if you use providers that belong to the plan's network. You may use doctors, hospitals, and providers outside of the network for an additional cost. You are typically not required to obtain a PCP. This type of plan is typically more expensive than other plans. It does allow the consumer more freedom in choosing providers and services.

Point-of-Service Plan (POS)

A point-of-service plan (POS) is a plan in which you pay less if you use doctors, hospitals, and other health care providers that belong to the plan's network. POS plans also require you to get a referral from your primary care doctor when seeing a specialist. POS plans typically will allow for out-of-network coverage. A POS plan is considered a cross between an HMO and PPO plan. Costs for a POS plan tend to run higher than an HMO or PPO plan.

Travel Medical Insurance

Medicare generally does not cover costs for medical care in a foreign country. Certain Medigap plans may cover international travel.

There are three options regarding travel insurance. Travel insurance is the type of coverage that covers your financial investment in your trip. It will cover lost baggage and canceled flights. It is *not* medical insurance and does not cover medical costs. Travel medical insurance may be purchased, and it covers foreign medical treatment and care. The last type of insurance is medical evacuation services; this insurance will provide coverage for air ambulance, medical evacuation, or medical escort service coverage for overseas travelers. The website travelstate.gov has a listing of U.S.-based companies that sell travel and medical insurance. As with any insurance product, it is best to fully understand what is covered and to what degree. The different insurance types are outlined in table 12.1.

TABLE 12.1   TYPES OF TRAVEL INSURANCE

Type	Coverage
Travel insurance	Baggage, flight cancellations
Travel medical insurance	Foreign medical care
Medical evacuation insurance	Air ambulance or medical evacuation

Source: U.S. Department of State, Bureau of Consular Affairs

CLINICAL PEARL

Durable medical equipment is covered under Medicare Part B. One example is a transcutaneous electrical nerve stimulation unit (TENS). TENS units can be helpful in reducing muscular or nerve-based pain. Medicare has traditionally reimbursed medical vendors up to $600 for such units. If your physician writes a prescription for a unit and the prescription is taken to a medical supply or equipment business, it may bill Medicare or your insurance company $800 for such a unit, leaving you with a copay of $200 or more. Very similar units can be purchased online for about $29–49 dollars. The cheaper units are effective. They can also save you a significant amount of money.

Resources

Centers for Medicare and Medicaid Services (CMS): Main homepage for the Medicare and Medicaid services; starting point for having your questions answered with numerous links exploring all aspects of the programs: https://www.cms.gov/

LBJ Presidential Library: Website to learn further perspectives on the history of Medicare and Medicaid and President Johnson's roles in the programs: http://www.lbjlibrary.org/

Chapter 13

The Internet and the World of Medicine

Traditionally physicians have embraced technology. New discoveries or techniques have been at the forefront of medical advancements. The internet is a technology that can both aid and inhibit the practice of medicine. The internet has enabled physicians to share a wealth of information including research studies, the latest techniques, and information presented at medical conferences. Potential negatives include patients' incorrect self-diagnosis and exploration of sites that are based on a commercial or business model rather than a medical one. This chapter will provide information and an understanding to assist consumers with use of the internet and the world of medicine.

Innovation

The internet is a technology that has affected many levels of medicine.[1] The internet has a plethora of unlimited information. Before the internet, patients would be seen in a doctor's office where they would be given a diagnosis and information. The information was communicated or provided to the patient in the forms of pamphlets or information sheets. The patient would accept the information given and then follow the instructions.

Today anyone can search the internet for medical information. Consumers can now visit many sites that inform and educate doctors. Popular search engines can be used to find scholarly journals, slide presentations, and clinical guidelines. Consumers and patients can also visit chat rooms and blogs. These sites can be beneficial in some cases and problematic in others.

Dr. Google

A great number of patients use the search engine Google to begin their search of symptoms to make a diagnosis of their medical problems. How accurate is such a practice? In terms of diagnostic accuracy this question was researched by two Australian specialists. They tested the diagnostic accuracy of Google searches by entering symptoms and signs from 26 published case records. The search revealed the correct diagnosis in 15 cases and the incorrect diagnosis in the remaining 11 cases.[2]

What can you possibly learn from your healthcare provider that is not available on the internet? Sir Francis Bacon is credited for the phrase "knowledge is power," which is very true, but it is important to know that knowledge is not wisdom. Given their extensive training, physicians and other healthcare providers are in the best position to weigh information and advise patients, drawing on their understanding of available evidence and their training and experience.[1]

When patients perform an online search of a disease, they will receive the search results. The results can sometimes be commercially influenced. The search will not differentiate from the most likely to the least likely possibilities. For example, if a consumer searches "low back and leg pain" the resulting terms will yield various sites and links. By clicking on the random link, the consumer may get locked into a less likely diagnosis of piriformis syndrome rather than the more likely lumbar disc as the cause of their leg pain. They may then search for treatments of the incorrect diagnosis, causing further delay in the appropriate treatment or the potential for worsening their current condition. The health care provider will then need to spend additional time convincing the patient of the correct diagnosis and dispelling the incorrect one.

Domains

The domain name is part of the uniform resource locator (URL) used to access websites. The top-level domain (TLD) name is located just to the right of the web address. Common TLD names include com, edu, gov, net, and org. The TLD name can assist the consumer in identifying the source and potential motives of each site.

The TLD ".gov" denotes a government site. This TLD can be the source of good health information. Sites that are sponsored by the federal government include the U.S. Department of Health and Human Services (www.hhs.gov), the FDA (www.fda.gov), the National Institutes of Health (www.nih.gov), the Centers for Disease Control and Prevention (www.cdc.gov), and the National Library of Medicine (www.nlm.nih.gov). All of these sites have updated information and are felt to be free of commercial bias.

The TLD ".edu" denotes an education site. They also are felt to be a very good sources of health information considering they are sites that are run by universities or medical schools. These sites will present medical information directed at informing the consumer and describing particular providers, centers, or clinics of the medical center that will address these certain problems.

Organizations are denoted by the TLD ".org." They also are good sources of health information. These sites are maintained by not-for-profit groups whose focus is research and teaching the public about specific diseases or conditions.

Quick question: What does the .com refer to? Answer: The TLD ".com" is short for commercial, commercial as in pertaining to a business or a product. These sites can appear to be both informative and impressive. It is always best to keep in mind that commercial sites and are also interested in *selling* products or services and will also contain ads. These sites may provide some medical information, but should be viewed with some caution.

Starting Point

You were just informed by your health care provider that you have multiple sclerosis. Now what? I would strongly recommend initiating your start to further investigate a medical condition or diagnosis to one of the sites listed. They all serve as a very good initial site to visit to commence education regarding a particular diagnosis.

Medlineplus.gov: This site is sponsored by the National Institutes of Health and is managed by the U.S. National Library of Medicine. MedlinePlus provides information on more than nine hundred diseases and conditions in their "Health Topics" section and links to other trusted resources. The links of specific organizations can further serve to educate and enhance the basic information.

MayoClinic.com: This page is operated by the Mayo Foundation for Medical Education and Research this site is produced by more than 3,300 physicians, scientists and researchers from Mayo Clinic. It provides in-depth, easy-to-understand information on hundreds of diseases and conditions, drugs and supplements, tests and procedures. It is a ".com" site, though in this case a good and trustworthy site.

Another good site for medical information is **healthfinder.gov**. This site is sponsored by the Office of Disease Prevention and Health Promotion within the U.S. Department of Health and Human Services. The site is intended for consumers and lists recommendations for preventative care based on gender and age. In addition, it has information on a number of health topics from A–Z.

Evidence-Based Medicine

Research is of vital importance to medicine. Research is done to further our understanding of what works and what does not work when it comes to treatments. Research and various outcomes serve to differentiate medicine from other industries or disciplines. The term *evidence-based medicine* (EBM) integrates clinical experience and patient values with the best available research information.[3] This research is based on the use of high-quality clinical research to guide treatments. EBM requires the physician to be skillful at both searching and interpreting research studies (literature). The literature may evaluate the effectiveness of a treatment, determine causality of a particular disease, or describe a potential new treatment approach.

Medical literature is comprised of medical journals, which contain articles, commentaries, and reviews that look to further advance our understanding of medicine. The articles may serve to review a medical topic, thoroughly discussing the current understanding of a disease. The article may describe the particular disease in terms of etiology (cause), diagnosis, and treatments. Other articles in medical journals may describe the results or a new or novel treatment focusing on the outcomes of such treatments. Commentaries will offer opinions on a particular topic and many consumers may be surprised to know that opinions on treatment approaches do not always achieve a 100-percent consensus among medical professionals.

Historically, medical journals have been published in a way that is similar to a magazine in terms of size and quality of the binding. Recently, journals are being accessed electronically more and more.

Research Studies

There are different types of research studies and the types fall under a hierarchy based on their level of importance. Not all research gets published. Certain scientific standards must typically be attained for a study to be published in a medical journal. Many journals will require a peer-review process. The editorial staff is made up of physicians, many of whom are leaders in their field of medicine. The journal may have the article "peer reviewed" by these physicians. This is the process that ensures a basic standard for published research.

There are different research studies that can be performed. Animal research, case report study, case control study, cohort study, randomized controlled trial (RTC), systematic review, and meta-analysis are the different types that will be reviewed. They will now be presented in the order from lesser to a greater level of evidence or significance. It is important for consumers to have a basic understanding of the different studies as the marketing departments will highlight the fact that their products have been "scientifically shown" to work. Positive results noted in an animal research study or a case report study are much different than positive results or proven effectiveness in a RTC or a meta-analysis.

Animal Research

Animals may be the initial testing focus for a novel device, medicine, or medical procedure. Testing on animals is done for the purpose of determining the effects of the potential treatment. For medicine testing, the emphasis will be on the effects of the medicine as well as its potential damage to the body (toxicology). Medicine testing will be performed on animals, and if no toxic effects are observed, it will then proceed to phase 1 testing on humans. The medical procedure of a bone marrow transplantation was initially performed on animals, before it was proven to be safe for humans. Researchers Dr. Joseph E. Murray and Dr. E. Donnall Thomas received the Noble prize in physiology or medicine in 1990 for their research. They were jointly awarded the prestigious award "for their discoveries concerning organ and cell transplantation in the treatment of human disease." This potential life-saving procedure of bone marrow transplantation, according to the HSRA is performed on an estimated 19,000 patients per year.[4]

Case Report Study

A case report study is a report that focuses on a single patient and his or her disease, treatment and outcome. The placebo response associated with pain relief is 30 percent, so this factor should be kept in mind. Additionally, different individuals can respond differently to medicines. The differences include both the medication's efficacy (success rate) and its side effects. The case report study is valuable in the sense that if a new treatment is successful and the article allows others to know of the treatment, further testing and investigation may be done to confirm the initial claims.

Case Control Study

A case control study is a research study that essentially works backward. The study will begin looking at a particular outcome or disease that has occurred in a group of individuals and then looks for potential causes. It will compare a group of individuals who have the disease with a group of individuals who do not have the disease. The study will then work backward (retrospectively) to find if a certain exposure is associated with the disease. For example, it may take a group of patients with colon cancer and compare them to a group of patients without colon cancer. Researchers will ask them both about their diet, specifically their intake of fats. The researchers may be able to then note that the group with a higher intake of saturated fat was four times more likely to develop colon cancer than the group that had a lower intake of saturated fat in their diet.

Cohort Study

A cohort study follows a group over an extended period of time and analyzes risk factors or exposures to determine who in the group develops a certain disease. This type of study is usually done on a prospective basis. The landmark cohort study is the Framingham Heart Study. This study was started in 1948 by a group of researchers looking to identify risk factors for heart disease. The study is still ongoing and sponsored by the National Heart, Blood, and Lung Institute and Boston University. The Framingham Heart

Study has immensely improved our understanding of heart disease and risk factors. According to the Framingham Heart Study, we now know the following: Cigarette smoking has been found to increase the risk of heart disease (1960), high blood pressure has been found to increase the risk of stroke (1970), high levels of HDL (good) cholesterol have been found to reduce the risk of death (1988), the progression from high blood pressure to heart failure was described (1996), and sleep apnea has been found to increase the risk of stroke (2010). This is an abbreviated list of the more than 33 significant findings that have been discovered in the Framingham Heart Study.

Randomized Control Trial (RCT)

A randomized control trial (RCT) is a study in which subjects are randomly chosen to receive one of several clinical interventions. The study is frequently done without subjects knowing the particular intervention that they are receiving, also known as a *blind RCT*. The strength of such research is in the randomization process. Physicians may also refer to this study as the gold standard. This refers to the fact that when the study is done correctly the conclusions are very convincing in terms of treatment efficacy (effectiveness). Examples of an RCT may be testing of a new medication for high blood pressure. The subjects are split into two groups: A and B. Group A is assigned the experimental medicine to lower blood pressure. Group B is assigned a placebo tablet (control group). Both groups do not know whether they are given the medicine or placebo tablet that will not affect blood pressure (blind RCT). Their blood pressure is monitored and recorded for three months. The results are analyzed for both groups. The researchers will determine if Group A had better control of their blood pressures with the experimental medicine compared to Group B, which received the placebo. The results can then be published, advancing the possible treatments for high blood pressure.

Systematic Review

A systematic review is a research paper that will summarize the results of previously published studies. The systematic review will typically summarize well-designed healthcare studies (controlled trials). When the studies are reviewed together, the collective results can provide a high level of evidence. This higher level of evidence can provide better clarity to the efficacy of the medications or interventions, allowing for better recommendations for physicians and healthcare providers. Cochrane is associated with performing systematic reviews. Cochrane is a global independent network of researchers, professionals, patients, caregivers, and people interested in health. According to their website, they have 37,000 contributors from more than 130 countries. They work together to produce credible, accessible health information that is free from commercial sponsorship and other conflicts of interest. The website also produces Cochrane reviews to achieve this goal, producing reviews on a variety of medically related topics.

Meta-Analysis

A meta-analysis is similar to a systematic review in that it combines previously published studies and reviews the results. The main difference is that the meta-analysis will incorporate a statistical procedure that integrates the results of several independent studies considered to be "combinable."[5] The meta-analysis will then statistically derive a conclusion based on the analysis. The meta-analysis can be beneficial since it includes a consolidated and quantitative review of a large, and often complex, sometimes apparently conflicting body of literature.[6] Given the extensive amount of ongoing research and the availability to search and review online, this type of study is now feasible.

Searches

Both health care professionals and consumers can search the medical literature online. MEDLINE is the U.S. National Library of Medicine® (NLM) premier bibliographic database. Remember that MEDLINE plus is a recommended site consumers should use as a starting point for learning more about a disease or diagnosis. MEDLINE is the primary component of PubMed (pubmed.gov); a link to PubMed is found on the NLM homepage (www.nlm.nih .gov). The result of a MEDLINE/PubMed search is a list of citations (including authors, title, source, and often an abstract) to journal articles and an indication of free electronic full-text availability. Searching is free of charge and does not require registration. A growing number of MEDLINE citations contain a link to the free full text of the article archived in Pub Med Central™ or to other sites.

Consumers can search terms to determine if research studies may support claims they have heard or read about. To begin a search one needs to enter the key words of the search into PubMed. For example, if one wants to know if green tea lowers risks of cancer, one would enter "green tea," "cancer," and "reduction" into the search. The result will show a number of studies in chronologic order (newest first). If one wishes to evaluate a study further, one would simply click on it. One will likely get an abstract (summary) of the study and a link to the entire study. For most consumers, reading of the abstract will likely be sufficient to answer their question. The articles are written in scientific language and may not be easy to understand, but the main point of the article will be summarized in fairly easy-to-understand language in the conclusion (last) section of the abstract. The method(s) section of the abstract will define the type of study and state the number of subjects involved. This will help to put the results in their proper perspective of significance when comparing the different types of research studies in the hierarchy of significance.

Claims

Snake oil salesmen have been around for centuries. These individuals may be easy to spot and consumers are very aware of their tactics. Claims on the internet may be harder to interpret. An internet site may have impressive graphics, seem official, or be associated with an organization. As mentioned before, TLD with ".com" denotes it as a commercial site and the intent of those running the site may be to sell a product rather than provide information to the consumer.

Be aware when a product claims, "one product does it all." The product may be promoted to help with heart disease, back pain, diabetes and cancer. Those disease processes are entirely different from one another and one medicine has not been scientifically proven to treat all of them. The aforementioned diagnoses do have one thing in common: They are the most commonly diagnosed conditions in the United States. These products also are supported by personal testimonies, but remember this is not considered an adequate form of medical evidence.

The term "natural" is often associated with safe. This is not always the case. Natural products can certainly be dangerous. Botulinum is produced by bacteria naturally and can be fatal if ingested, and rattlesnake venom is also natural. If a product was a cure for a serious disease, it would be widely reported in the media. It would then be regularly prescribed by health professionals. The miracle product would not be found in a magazine or newspaper ad, late-night television show, or infomercial.

Quick fixes are also a concerning claim. Unfortunately, cancer cannot be eliminated in a few days with any product at this time. The gimmicky cures will usually target the individuals with chronic pain or a diagnosis with limited medical treatments. The claims may also involve paranoid accusations in an attempt to gain one's support or belief in the product. Examples may include the following catch phrase, "Get the all-natural cure the drug companies are trying to hide." These types of claims suggest that healthcare providers and legitimate manufacturers are partnering to promote their products for a mutual financial gain.

The internet can be a source of good medical information. The techniques outlined in this chapter should equip the consumer with the necessary skills to navigate the internet appropriately and safely with respect to medicine.

CLINICAL PEARL

Consumers (patients) need to be somewhat cautious in regards to chat rooms. Chat rooms can at times be helpful in obtaining a better understanding of a disease, illness, or sickness. The understanding can come from one person relating his or her experiences of a particular disease. His or her experiences can help other patients to provide them with a better understanding of the disease, and it can give them a better understanding of what symptoms and potential course of the disease to expect. Caution is advised when it comes to treatments. Patients may tout various treatments or reference healthcare providers who provided miraculous cures. These patients may be individuals who truly do not have the disease and are providing false information in an attempt to sell a product or influence a potentially desperate (hoping to find a cure/treatment) patient to a certain healthcare provider.

Resources

Cochrane: Homepage for Cochrane, a group of researchers who examine the evidence and allow for informed decisions regarding medical treatments from their statistical reviews: http://www.cochrane.org/about-us

Framingham Heart Study: Website for the long-running research study and efforts of Boston University and the National Heart, Lung, and Blood Institute: https://www.framinghamheartstudy.org/

National Library of Medicine: Home of the National Library of Medicine, with links for Pub Med, Medline plus, toxic information, and clinical trials: https://www.nlm.nih.gov/

Endnotes

1. Pamela Hartzband and Jerome Groopman, "Untangling the Web—Patients, Doctors, and the Internet," *New England Journal of Medicine* 362 (2010):1063–1066.
2. Hangwi Tang and Jennifer Hwee Kwoon Ng, "Googling for a Diagnosis—Use of Google as a Diagnostic Aid: Internet Based Study," *BMJ* 333 (2006): 1143–1145.
3. Izet Masic, Milan Miokovic, and Belma Muhamedagic, "Evidence Based Medicine: New Approaches and Challenges," *Acta Informatica Medica* 16, no. 4 (2008): 219–25.
4. "Transplant Activity Report," *Health Resources and Services Administration*, https://bloodcell.transplant.hrsa.gov/research/transplant_data/transplant_activity_report/index.html
5. Matthias Egger, George Davey Smith, and Andrew N. Phillips, "Meta-Analysis: Principles and Procedures," *BMJ* 315 (1997): 1533–7.
6. Anna-Bettina Haidich, "Meta-Analysis in Medical Research," *Hippokratia* 14, no. 1 (2010): 29–37.

Chapter 14

Long-Term Care and End-of-Life Issues

As Benjamin Franklin once said, "Our new Constitution is now established, everything seems to promise it will be durable; but, in this world, nothing is certain except death and taxes." Similarly, both aging and death are a part of life. The idea of death can be difficult to think about and potentially plan for. The initial part of this chapter will discuss long-term care in terms of both planning and options consumers have, while the latter half will address end-of-life issues.

Long-Term Care

Long-term care includes a number of services and supports that people may need to meet their personal care needs. Most long-term care is *not* true medical care, but rather assistance with basic personal tasks of everyday life, known as activities of daily living (ADLs). ADLs may include bathing, dressing, using the toilet, transfers, and eating. These are skills that most of us take for granted, but ones that can be a challenge in elderly individuals with underlying medicine problems such as arthritis, stroke, or memory deficits (dementia).

The U.S. Department of Health and Human Services (HHS) estimates that 70 percent of Americans older than 65 will require some level of long-term care. What factors play a role in determining who is more likely to require long-term care? One of these factors is age. As one ages the likelihood of requiring care increases. Of the current population receiving long-term care, 3.6 million (37 percent) were under age 65 and 6 million (63%) were over age 65.[1] Gender also plays a role, with women having a five-year greater life expectancy than men. Governmental statistics show that women need care longer on average (3.7 years) than men (2.2 years). If you live alone, you are more likely to need paid care than if you are married or living with someone.

Caregivers

The HHS estimates that about 80 percent of care at home is provided by unpaid caregivers, often family members who spend about spend twenty hours a week giving care. More than half (58 percent) have intensive caregiving responsibilities that may include assisting with an ADL. In the majority of cases most adults may be able to live at home for many years with a combination of support from family, friends, and paid caregivers. When the care of an individual exceeds what can be provided in the home, there is a wide array of services, centers, and programs available.

Costs

The costs associated with the level of care also vary considerably. According to HHS the cost averages can range from $21 per hour for a home health aide, $67 per day for an adult day care center, and $229 per day for a private room in a nursing home. The costs are outlined in table 14.1. The costs can also vary depending on the geographic region of the country one lives in.

TABLE 14.1 NATIONAL AVERAGES OF LONG-TERM CARE COSTS

Level of Care	Costs
Homemaker services	$20 per hour
Home health aide	$21 per hour
Adult day care	$68 per day
Assisted living facility	$3,628 per month
Semi-private room in nursing home	$6,844 per month
Private room in nursing home	$7,698 per month

According to HHS 2016

How to Pay for Long-Term Care

Medicare does not typically pay or cover long-term care beyond a short period of time, and it is dependent on certain conditions being met. Medicare will pay for long-term care if one requires skilled services or rehabilitative care. Medicare will cover care in a nursing home for a maximum of 100 days and this usually follows an inpatient hospitalization for a new medical problem or diagnosis.

Medicaid does pay for the largest share of long-term care services. Medicaid is the federal insurance place for the poor that is administered at the state level. In order to qualify for Medicaid your income and assets must be below a certain level. Congress passed the Deficit Reduction Act of 2005. This act has a look-back period of five years to examine an individual's assets to determine Medicaid eligibility. This act was passed in order to increase the look-back period from three years to five years. It was done to prevent fraud and limit the ability to allow financially wealthy individuals to transfer all of their assets to their children and then be eligible for free long-term nursing care.

Health insurance, either employer sponsored or private health insurance (including health insurance plans), provide benefits, and coverage is similar to the coverage of Medicare, which can be limited. Insurance may cover long-term care, though it is typically only for skilled, short-term, medically necessary care. There are an increasing number of private payment options including long-term care insurance, reverse mortgages, life insurance options, and annuities that can fund long-term care costs.

Buying Long-Term Care Insurance

Long-term care insurance is private insurance. It is important to keep in mind that individuals with certain pre-existing health conditions may not qualify for long-term insurance. For this reason, it is recommended to purchase long-term care insurance well before you may need to use it.

One may not be eligible to purchase the insurance based on pre-existing conditions. Some conditions include AIDS, any form of dementia, a history of a stroke, and certain cancers. Insurance companies also consider other health conditions when determining your eligibility, but if you buy your long-term care insurance before you develop one of the health conditions listed, then your policy will cover the care you need for that condition.

It costs less to buy coverage when you are younger, so one can lock into a lower premium or rate, which may provide savings and longer coverage long term. The average age that people buy into long-term care insurance today is about 60 years old. It is also important to know what specific types of long-term care are covered with the current policy being offered or potentially acquired.

Types of Long-Term Care

The different levels of long-term care are based on the needs of the individual and range from community support services to nursing facilities with 24-hour supervision. If specialized care is required, a nurse, home health or home care aide, and/or therapist may provide care at the house. This type of care may be covered by Medicare on a short-term basis.

Adult Day Care

Community services are support services that can include adult day care, meal programs, senior centers, transportation, and other services. These can help people who are cared for at home and by their families. For example, adult day care services provide a variety of health, social, and related support services in a protective setting during the day. Often these individuals return home in the evening, with supervision then being provided by their working adult children. This service can be helpful for elderly adults with impairments that affect memory and cognition (Alzheimer's disease or dementia). The services can also provide the at-home caregiver with a much-needed break or respite.

Home Care Services

Home care services are regulated at the state level and must be licensed. Consumers can check with their state health department to determine if the home care agency is licensed. Agencies may also be certified at the federal level by Medicare. Medicare will perform home health care agency inspections to assure they meet certain standards by federal health and safety requirements. Medicare will only pay for services if the agency is certified by Medicare.

The public can determine if the home health care agency is certified by Medicare by reviewing its survey report. The consumer will need to call the Medicare hotline at 1-800-633-4227 and ask for the home health hotline for their state. One can then request a copy of the home health report from that hotline. In addition, one can determine if the agency has been accredited (awarded a "seal of approval") by a group such as the Joint Commission on Accreditation of Healthcare Organizations (630-792-5800; http://www.jcaho.org) or the Community Health Accreditation Program (1-800-669-1656; http://www.chapinc.org).

In addition, one can always contact his or her state consumer affairs office to see if any complaints have been filed against a particular home care agency. References from other families or patients who have worked with the agency can also be requested. Consumers may also request to see the certifications or licensure of the particular caregivers that will be coming into the house. By investigating ahead of time, poor outcomes can be avoided.

Nursing Home Factors to Consider

There are a number of factors to consider when choosing a nursing home for a loved one. Unfortunately, the cost of the facility will play a major role in the decision. An important factor to consider is when a senior spends down his or her life savings at a nursing home and then qualifies for Medicaid; will the nursing home accept Medicaid as a form of payment? If they do not, your loved one may need to be moved to another facility. The quality of the nursing home facility should also be a strong determining factor. The nursing home may be a new facility with high-end common space areas and décor, but is this at the expense of proper staffing? While a 65-inch flat screen television can serve to provide a favorable impressive on the tour of the facility, there are other significant factors to consider.

An important factor to consider is the certified staff to resident ratio. Find out if the facility is able to provide one-to-one care if necessary. Staff longevity is another factor to inquire about. High staff turnover may be associated with the staff feeling overwhelmed, overworked, and the facility being understaffed.

One can also inquire about activities that are available to the residents. Another clue may be the appearance of the residents: Are they well groomed and appropriately dressed? The cleanliness of the facility can also give an indication of the type of care provided. Are there strong odors or urine present? One may also consider the facilities' policy on having pets visit. It may be helpful to consider what factors are important to the family and devise a checklist prior to visiting a facility so these factors can be properly assessed.

Review Public Information

As of January 2003, all Medicaid- and Medicare-certified nursing homes are required to publicly post the number of nursing staff they have on duty each daily shift. Licensed and unlicensed staff include registered nurses, licensed practical nurses, and certified nursing aides. Nursing homes must also have the name and contact information for all state client advocacy agencies, the Medicaid fraud control unit, along with the results of the most recent state or federal survey. The state inspection report is available on Caregiverlist.com. It is based on an inspection every 15 months.

Advance Directives

An advanced directive, as defined by the National Cancer Institute, is a legal document that allows you to make known your decisions about end-of-life care ahead of time. The advance directive may include a living will and a durable power of attorney for health care. The advance directive document only goes into effect if you are incapacitated and unable to speak for yourself.

Living Will

A living will is a written document that communicates to your doctors how you want to be treated if you are dying or permanently unconscious and cannot make decisions about emergency treatments. The living will states in writing your choices in regards to CPR, artificial ventilation, artificial nutrition, dialysis, and certain medications.

Durable Power of Attorney for Health Care

Durable power of attorney of health care is a legal document naming a healthcare proxy. A proxy is an individual appointed to make medical decisions for you at times when you might not be able to do so. The proxy should be familiar with your values and wishes. This means that he or she will be able to decide which medical treatments and decisions will be made on your behalf.

Additional Advance Care

The do not resuscitate (DNR) order informs the medical staff in a hospital or nursing facility that you do not want them to try to return your heart to a normal rhythm if it stops or is in an unstable rhythm. Even though a living will might state CPR is not wanted, it is helpful to have a DNR order as part of your medical file if you go to a hospital. Posting a DNR next to your bed will help to avoid confusion in an emergency situation.

Cardiopulmonary Resuscitation (CPR)

Cardiopulmonary resuscitation (CPR) refers to treatments that may be employed in an attempt to restore a normal heart rhythm after an individual collapses, secondary to problems of the heart. These problems may occur when the heart is not able to beat in a normal matter. The heart may be beating at an irregular, extremely high rate, or in an uncoordinated fashion (fibrillations). In either case, the heart output is not sufficient to sustain life and constitutes a medical emergency.

CPR typically involves performing chest compressions on a collapsed victim. The chest is compressed in an attempt to deliver blood from the heart to the other areas of the body. Recently, there has been more emphasis placed on chest compressions and less on mouth-to-mouth resuscitation.

The other aspect of CPR focuses on restoring the heart rhythm. This can be done with the use of an automated external defibrillator (AED). AEDs can be identified by readily available signs. Their presence in public spaces, including arenas, gyms, and malls has been increasing. Research has shown that the sooner CPR can be started, the better the outcome. CPR has been found to be effective if started within four to six minutes from the time of the collapse and must be followed within 10–12 minutes of the collapse with advanced life support.[2]

Ventilator

A ventilator may be referred to as a breathing machine. This medical device will regulate breathing to ensure adequate oxygenation. The patient using a ventilator will be connected to the machine with a tube. The tube connects the machine to the patient's trachea or windpipe. The ventilator will force oxygenated air into the lungs. The process of having a tube placed into the trachea is uncomfortable, and most patients will require sedation via medications while on the ventilator.

Artificial Nutrition

If patients are unable to eat food safely, a feeding tube may be inserted. Patients recovering from a stroke or a head injury may require a feeding tube to provide adequate nutrition during their recovery. These measures can be helpful if one is recovering from an illness. Initially, the feeding tube is threaded through the nose down to the stomach. If supplemental feeding is needed for a longer time, then a gastric tube can be placed. This is usually by a gastroenterologist who surgically inserts the tube directly from the stomach and out to the skin surface. The tube provides easy access for nutrition, medications, and fluids. If the tube is no longer needed, it can be removed easily.

Artificial Hydration

When an individual is unable to drink water or swallow liquids, he or she can receive fluids via an intravenous (IV) route. The fluids and medications will be provided via an IV. This involves placing a small plastic tube (catheter) into a vein. The IV is usually placed into a vein in the hand or arm (commonly in the forearm area) to provide fluid when a person is unable to take in fluid orally (by mouth). Medications can also be given via an IV route. The fluid is usually supplied in a clear bag and hung on a pole. The IV route uses gravity to introduce the fluid into the body. The IV sites need to be rotated and changed every few days to lower the risk of a skin infection.

Comfort Care

Comfort care is done to soothe and relieve suffering while following the patient's wishes. It may include managing shortness of breath, offering ice chips for dry mouth, placing limits on medical testing, providing medications for pain or anxiety, and providing emotional support. The emotional support may be in the form of spiritual and emotional counseling.

Hospice care is intended to provide comfort to you and your family during a life-threatening illness rather than provide treatments to cure the illness. Hospice care does not imply no care and usually utilizes comfort care measures. It generally does not include additional diagnostic testing.

Palliative care differs from hospice care in that it is offered along with any medical treatments you might be receiving for a life-threatening illness. The tenets of both hospice and palliative care are to keep the patient comfortable. It is important to keep in mind that one can always move from hospice to palliative care if one wants to pursue treatments during his or her illness.

Physician Orders for Life-Sustaining Treatment (POLST)

Some states make use of a POLST. This order is intended for people who have already been diagnosed with a serious illness. This form does not replace a patient's advance directives. It serves as doctor-ordered instructions to ensure that, in case of an emergency, you receive the treatment you prefer. The POLST is posted near your bed, where emergency personnel or other medical team members can easily find it. The doctor will fill out the form based on the contents of your directives, discussions with your doctor about the likely course of the illness, and your treatment preferences.

CLINICAL PEARL

If you suffer a cardiac arrest in the United States, which city has the best survival rate? The answer is Seattle, Washington. According to King County EMS, someone who has a cardiac arrest in King County has a greater chance of survival than anyone else in the world, according the latest analysis by county officials. The survival rate for cardiac arrest in King County hit an all-time high of

62 percent in 2013. By comparison, the cardiac survival rates in New York City, Chicago, and other urban areas have been recorded to be in the single digits.

Seattle is able to have this remarkable distinction for a number of reasons. They have adopted high-performance CPR methods by emergency medical technicians in order to maximize oxygen circulation and increase survival chances. The county also utilizes telecommunications CPR, whereby 911 emergency personnel provide instant CPR instructions by phone. The city has prioritized the increasing public availability of automated external defibrillators (AEDs). Local residents also have very high rates of CPR training. Lastly, they support a regional paramedic training program, funded by charitable contributions, that exceeds national standards for certification. Emphasis is at all levels to improve outcomes.

Resources

LongTermCare.gov: U.S. Department of Health and Human services site with specific page on the basics of long-term care: https://longtermcare .acl.gov/the-basics/index.html

Medicare.gov: Web page with information on long-term care and links to assist with identifying appropriate care providers and facilities: https://www.medicare.gov/coverage/long-term-care.html

The Joint Commission: Web page that outlines the role of the joint commission as well as links to determine a facilities current accreditation status: https://www.jointcommission.org/

Community Health Accreditation Partner: Homepage of an agency that works to accredit home health agencies and can serve as a resource in identifying these agencies: http://www.chapinc.org/what-we-do/chap-accreditation.aspx

Elder Care: U.S. agency of aging sponsored site that allows for consumers to identify specific long-term services for their particular location by entering their zip code: http://www.eldercare.gov

Endnotes

1. S. Rogers and H. Komisar, "Who Needs Long-Term Care? Fact Sheet: Long-Term Care Financing Project," Georgetown University, Washington, DC (2003).
2. Richard O. Cummins, Mickey S. Eisenberg, Alfred P. Hallstrom, and Paul E. Litwin, "Survival of Out-of Hospital Cardiac Arrest with Early Initiation of Cardiopulmonary Resuscitation," *American Journal of Emergency Medicine* 3, no. 2 (1985): 114–9.

CPSIA information can be obtained
at www.ICGtesting.com
Printed in the USA
FSHW011734230719
60322FS